MW00837952

INTERMITTENT FASTING
FOR WOMEN OVER 50

A Perfect Guide to Losing Weight, Reset Your Metabolism, Boost Your Energy and Eating Healthy with 60+ Recipes and 21 Days Meal Plan

KAT WILDMAN

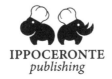

IPPOCERONTE
publishing

Copyright © 2021 by Kat Wildman
All rights reserved.

This document is geared towards providing exact and reliable information about the topic and issue covered. The publication is sold with the idea that the publisher is not required to render accounting, officially permitted, or otherwise, qualified services. If advice is necessary, legal, or professional, a practiced individual in the profession should be ordered.

From a Declaration of Principles which was accepted and approved equally by a Committee of the American Bar Association and a Committee of Publishers and Associations.

In no way is it legal to reproduce, duplicate, or transmit any part of this document in either electronic means or printed format. Recording of this publication is strictly prohibited, and any storage of this document is not allowed unless with the written permission from the publisher. All rights reserved.

The information provided herein is stated to be truthful and consistent, in that liability, in terms of inattention or otherwise, by any usage or abuse of any policies, processes, or directions contained within is the solitary and utter responsibility of the recipient reader. Under no circumstances will any legal responsibility or blame be held against the publisher for any reparation, damages, or monetary loss due to the information herein, either directly or indirectly.

Respective authors own all copyrights not held by the publisher.

The information herein is offered for informational purposes solely and is universal as s0. The presentation of the information is without a contract or any type of guaranteed assurance.

The trademarks that are used are without any consent, and the publication of the trademark is without permission or backing by the trademark owner.
All trademarks and brands within this book are for clarifying purposes only and are owned by the owners themselves, not affiliated with this document.

Book Formatting designed by macrovector / Freepik and thiwwy design,
Cover designed by thiwwy design (@thiwwy)

∽ CONTENT ∾

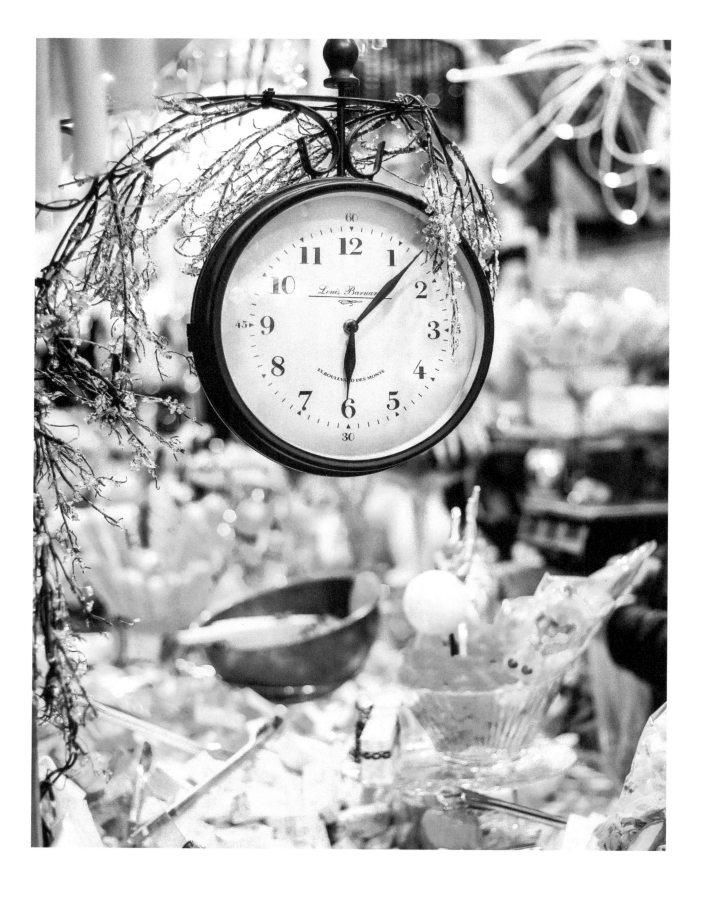

∽ INTRODUCTION ∾

Throughout our life, our body is in constant transformation. Men and women typically reach their physical peak in their late 20's to early 30's. After this time, muscle mass, strength, and flexibility begin to decline. Becoming aware of these changes could be scary at first, but there are various ways to slow down the natural decline of our body and stay in good physical and mental shape.

The first step to improving our fitness is accepting that our body responds differently to diets and fitness based on various factors, including age. From a young age, metabolism has not been my best friend; I've always had trouble staying fit, and any excess eating immediately turned into a few extra pounds. The difficulties in accepting my body prompted me to become interested in nutrition and then graduate in food science abroad in Rome.

My studies helped me understand and accept my body; it also taught me that there is no magic diet that works for everyone. Many people talk about the Keto diet or Sirt food diet as foolproof solutions to solve any weight problem. But, unfortunately, the real world doesn't work that way, and what is effective for one person may not work for another. Intermittent Fasting techniques are also no exception.

A diet to be effective must consider many factors, including age; for this reason, all the techniques presented in this book are designed for people over 50 who want to lose those extra pounds simply and safely. What a lot of diet books are not taking into account is the age factor. This is one of the many factors that can dramatically influence the results of a diet and can represent the difference between my clients' frustration and success.

Many women, as they age, experience reduced metabolism. Unfortunately, I have been there, and you might be in the same situation. The best way to correct this is by resetting your metabolism, which is precisely what Intermittent Fasting does. For those unfamiliar with the concept of metabolism, we will address this topic in more detail in the followings chapters. For now, think about metabolism as the way that your body uses food for energy.

This book aims to make available to the reader all the knowledge I have acquired in years of studying and work with my clients. I do not promise and never will promise miracles, but I am sure that once you learn the basics of Intermittent Fasting and the right mindset, you will get the long-lasting results you are looking for. I'm going to be honest with you, the journey we are about to embark on will not be easy at first; it will require time and the right level of commitment, but it will change your life.

Let's begin!

∽ CHAPTER 1 ∾

WHAT HAPPENS TO WOMEN'S BODIES AFTER 50

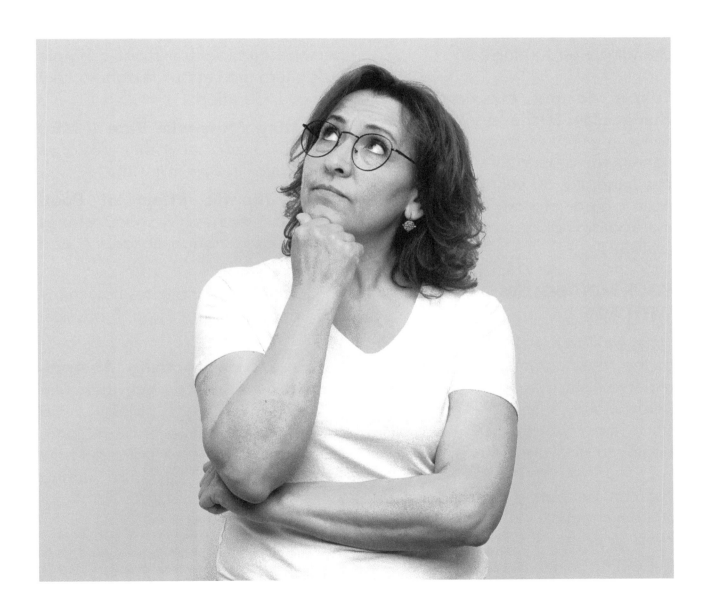

Usually, at this point, a diet book begins to describe the basics of a miraculous method that will change your life forever. I will not do anything like that, and I want to reiterate that there are no miraculous methods that work for everyone. So instead, I want to start talking about how our body changed after turning 50.

People do not experience these changes all at the same time. For some, it will have started a few years earlier, for others a few years later, but generally, 50 years is considered a turning point for our physiology and metabolism. Okay, so what's different after 50?

YOUR METABOLISM SLOWS DOWN WITH AGE

"I have a slow metabolism!" this is one of the most common excuses when a person starts to gain weight, but unfortunately, it is true in some cases since, as you age, your metabolism begins to slow down.

We can define your metabolism as all the chemical reactions that help keep your body active. A person's metabolism determines how many calories are consumed each day. Lucky people with a faster metabolism will burn calories faster than others, gaining weight much less easily. If you are reading this book, you are probably among ordinary people with a standard or slow speed metabolism. Although measuring how fast a person's metabolism is not a simple task, there are various factors to take into consideration:

- **Resting Metabolic Rate (RMR):** This indicates how many calories you burn in a resting state.

- **The Thermic Effect of Food (TEF):** indicates how many calories you burn through absorbing and digesting food.

- **Exercise:** This indicates how many calories you burn through physical activity.

- **Non-exercise Activity Ahermogenesis (NEAT):** Activities like walking, moving objects, and washing dishes still burn some calories. This index indicates how many calories you burn during these activities.

So, what are the main reasons why our metabolism slows down with age?

- **Less physical activity:** Physical exercise activities contribute 10% to 30% to the total calories burned daily. For some very active, people this number can reach even 50%! Unfortunately, research shows that older people tend to be less active than younger and over a quarter of Americans aged 50-65 don't do any physical activity outside work.

- **Our body is less efficient since its components are aging:** RMR is determined by two cellular components that drive chemical reactions inside our body. These components are called mitochondria and sodium-potassium pumps. According to various research papers, both components lose efficiency as we age, reducing daily burned calories.

- **As we age, we tend to lose lean muscle mass:** It has been estimated that the average adult can lose up to 8% of lean muscle mass during each decade (after 30). This process is known as sarcopenia and can lead to various health issues like fractures, weakness, and early death.

Sarcopenia also has the secondary effect of slowing down your metabolism since the amount of muscles mass increases your RMR. Sarcopenia happens for various reasons:

- Fewer calories and proteins are consumed during the day

- Hormone production is decreased (Estrogen, Testosterone, Growth Hormone)

- Reduced physical activity.

Having learned some of the basics of how metabolism works, your next question might be, "Okay, how much slower is my metabolism?"

There is no easy answer; there are various research papers on the argument, and the results obtained with the multiple experiments differ enormously in some cases.

All scientists seem to agree that the RMR tends to decrease according to the age group, having found only one experiment to produce conflicting results on the subject. This latest experiment followed a group of people for decades by measuring their metabolism. It has been hypothesized that the minimal variation of RMR found during this experiment is due to the extreme longevity of some participants (over 95 years old). The underlying idea is that their unique metabolism was one of the main factors in increasing their longevity.

HGH PRODUCTION IS LOWER

Human Growth Hormone (HGH) is an important hormone produced by our pituitary gland, and it plays a critical role in various instances:

- Muscle growth
- Body composition
- Cell repair
- Metabolism
- Body strength
- Physical exercise performance
- Injury and diseases recovery

As you can imagine, a reduction in the production of this hormone can directly affect the quality of our life and facilitate weight gain. The scientific community believes that there is a direct correlation between HGH levels and fat mass percentage in our bodies.

After monitoring the HGH release levels of more than a thousand patients over 24 hours, a considerable decline was observed in patients with the highest belly fat percentage. Unfortunately, the decline in HGH production is not mainly determined by body dysfunctions but most commonly by aging. There are **various ways to improve our HGH production**, the most common is to start an appropriate Intermittent Fasting diet.

Through appropriate intermittent Fasting is possible to raise HGH levels by over 300% in only three days. While progressing with the diet, the levels of HGH production will continue to rise until reaching 1250% after one week. We will talk more about the IF diet in the following chapters; for now, it is essential to remember that some type of Intermittent Fasting is not meant for long periods and should be stopped at the most opportune moment.

Another way to increase HGH levels is assuming supplements, *Arginine* and *GABA (Gamma-aminobutyric acid)*, are usually the two most popular choices. However, it is important to note that recent studies show that the best results are found while also doing physical activity. Therefore, supplements alone might not sort the desired effect.

Eating in a controlled manner can help improve HGH levels. For example, reducing the daily sugar intake will help reduce the insulin levels in our bodies. This will consequently facilitate the production of HGH.

It also plays a fundamental role when we eat our meals; having a late dinner, especially if rich in carbohydrates, will increase our insulin levels by inhibiting the nocturnal production of HGH.

It is therefore advisable to **have dinner no later than 3 hours before going to bed**.

HIT (High-Intensity Training) is another effective way to raise your HGH levels. Physical exercise, in general, plays a crucial role in improving your HGH production. Studies have shown that HIT is the type of exercise that has the most significant impact on HGH production. The peak of HGH production occurs during the night when our body is at rest. We can visualize the release of HGH as pulses coordinated by our internal clock – Circadian Rhythm. Since most HGH is released before midnight, studies have shown that a poor sleep schedule can be one of the leading causes of the reduction of HGH levels.

Optimizing our sleep, therefore, plays a fundamental role; the perfect rest can be obtained with some simple changes in your lifestyle:

- Avoid caffeine and sugars before going to bed.
- Do relaxing activities, such as reading a book, when in bed.
- Make sure your bedroom is quiet and at a comfortable temperature.
- Avoid blue light exposure before bedtime – such as the one generated by smartphones.

With aging, it is not easy to maintain optimal levels of HGH; for this reason, it is possible to resort to various **supplements** that can help us in this task:

- *Creatine*: It can help increasing HGH levels for 2-6 hours.
- Glycine: According to some *studies*, it can help with short-term spikes in HGH. Your doctor might suggest it to better support physical activity.
- *Glutamine*: It can help to raise HGH levels up to 80% - temporarily.
- *L-dopa*: This is used mainly for Parkinson's disease treatments and also helps to raise HGH levels.

I strongly suggest consulting a doctor before taking substances aimed at improving your HGH levels. It is always a good idea to discuss your case with a specialist to understand if you require one of these supplements and define the most appropriate dosage.

OTHER EFFECTS OF AGING

In this section, I would like to quickly provide an overview of the other effects of aging that impact our physical condition after 50.

Women's bones increase in density until the age of 30 but, after 35, we slowly begin to **lose bones' density** due to changes in hormone levels. This process of loss of density becomes even faster after menopause. No ways have been discovered yet to stop this constant decay, but it is possible to enormously slow it down with a healthy lifestyle and regular physical activity. For prevention purposes, it is also advisable to carry out a bones density screening exam around 50 to assess the situation and put into action the most appropriate remedies to fight osteoporosis years before the problem arises.

Unfortunately, **heart disease rates tend to rise after menopause**; this is due to the reduction in estrogen production. Estrogen helps keep arteries healthy and improves HDL levels, also known as "good cholesterol," while maintaining LDL under control known as "bad cholesterol."

After menopause, the amount of estrogen in our body begins to drop, increasing the risk of cardiovascular disease by up to 300%. Fortunately, there are methods to reduce this risk considerably; a balanced diet and regular exercise are, once again, our primary weapons in the fight against aging. In addition, as we will see later, Intermittent Fasting is a perfect method to reset our bodies and reduce the amount of LDL.

Unfortunately, you may have already noticed that aging does not even spare our skin and hair. Our skin begins to lose its elasticity after 40, and some annoying wrinkles start to appear. In addition, our hair becomes finer, less resistant, and prone to graying. Some of you may have noticed the first white hair already around the age of 30, while others, many years later. The graying of the hair is directly related to our genes, and it is a process that varies enormously from person to person. For all the effects not directly related to our genes, there are numerous ways to slow down the effects of aging but, there is no magic formula other than diet, physical training, and supplements.

As a woman reaches her forties and fifties, she goes through menopause; her hormones gradually decrease as her ovaries stop producing estrogen and progesterone, preventing menstruation. She is said to have entered menopause because she has not had a cycle for 12 months, but amenorrhea isn't the only symptom of menopause.

After menopause, women may become less receptive to insulin, as if the other signs weren't enough. As a result, they may have difficulty absorbing sugar and processed carbohydrates; this physiologic transition is known as insulin resistance, associated with fatigue, sleep difficulties, and weight gain.

As you will soon discover on your body, Intermittent Fasting is one of the most powerful allies we have in fighting the signs of aging; it is not only valuable for losing weight but also to reset our organism.

~ CHAPTER 2 ~

INTERMITTENT FASTING FOR WOMEN OVER 50

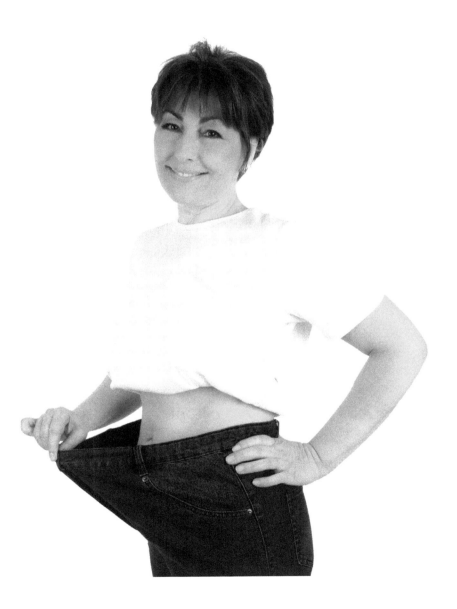

It is becoming increasingly more challenging for a woman to lose weight after the age of 50, and we're obsessed with those extra pounds that pile up in places we don't want them to, such as hips and love handles. Intermittent Fasting is a diet that differs from traditional diets, considering the numerous health and mental benefits of calorie restriction can also become a way of life. The various intermittent fasting types allow us to assess and select the best one for us, tailoring it to our specific needs and lifestyle. Before considering starting this type of diet, it is advisable to consult your doctor. Intermittent Fasting is a diet that, if carried out correctly, does not involve risks. Still, it is essential for more sensitive individuals or individuals with previous conditions to have an evaluation by a specialist.

INTERMITTENT FASTING IN A NUTSHELL

Intermittent Fasting is a way to lose weight by consuming calories during a short period. The daily intake is severely restricted, and the 24-hour fast is interrupted by periods of eating. For example, some people only eat from 12 noon until 8 pm, which is called the "lean gains method" after the fitness website on which it's promoted, while others stop eating after 6 pm—which is generally known as "16:8".

Intermittent Fasting has been around for a long time, and different variants of the method have emerged over time. It works by balancing your eating window with periods of fasting to regulate your blood sugar levels. After completing a fast, most people report feeling more energized, allowing them to increase their physical activity. In addition, you will have better insulin sensitivity and blood sugar control after doing intermittent Fasting.

Fasting for short periods is believed to help your metabolism, but not in the way you might think. IF does not speed up your metabolism; instead, it increases the efficiency of burning calories since the body is forced to adjust to extreme calorie restriction during an intermittent fasting session.

So basically, Intermittent Fasting not only affects your metabolism but can also aid in weight loss. When you go without food for a long time, your body starts to burn more fat and less muscle. As a result, you'll begin to lose weight as your body begins to remove fat from your tissues to conserve energy for other functions.

BENEFITS AND RISKS OF INTERMITTENT FASTING FOR WOMEN OVER 50

During my career, I have not tried to hide the negative aspects of a method, and I believe it is essential that you make an informed choice about a diet that could affect your future lifestyle. For this reason, before discussing the various intermittent fasting techniques in detail, I would like to explain the benefits and risks of adopting Intermittent Fasting.

Adopting intermittent Fasting can bring the following benefits:

- **Insulin levels:** The insulin level in the blood tends to drop, reducing the risk of type 2 diabetes.

- **HGH:** The production of HGH (Human Grown Hormone) increases, bringing a series of benefits, including ease in burning fat and acquiring greater muscle mass.

- **Cellular repair:** The purification deriving from IF facilitates the re-placement and repair of damaged cells giving new life to our organism.

- **Lose weight and visceral fat:** This happens since IF works on both sides of the calorie equation, boosting your metabolic rate and reducing the amount of food you consume.

- **Oxidative damage and inflammation:** Several studies show that IF may enhance the body's resistance to oxidative stress and help fight inflammation.

- **Hearth health:** IF improves various risk factors that might cause heart diseases; among these, we find: blood sugar levels, blood pressure, triglycerides, bad cholesterol, and inflammatory markers.

- **Alzheimer's prevention:** Various studies have shown that adopting an IF lifestyle can improve Alzheimer's symptoms. Also, animal studies are showing that Fasting might offer a certain level of protection against neurodegenerative diseases.

Potential Risk of Intermittent Fasting for women over 50:

- **Extreme Hunger:** IF requires some adaptation time for your body. The first few days of this diet are usually the most traumatic for some individuals.

- **Stress hormone:** IF may lead, in certain subjects, to increase cortisol production, causing increased stress and food cravings.

- **Overeating and binge eating:** I have seen in some of my clients overeating and binge eating behaviors. These are obviously highly harmful and could frustrate the efforts made.

- **Dehydration:** While getting used to this new lifestyle, some people tend to forget about drinking during fasting times. This, of course, is highly discouraged

- **Tiredness:** Consuming fewer calories means having less energy available. Especially in an initial period of adaptation, people who adopt IF feel tired and, in some cases, irritable (**mood swings**).

Intermittent Fasting is not for everyone and carries risks if not done correctly; *most of the problems that may* *arise from adopting IF can be solved by carefully following these few tips:*

- **Malnutrition** may sound frightening, but you can avoid it for the most part by eating well-balanced meals during your eating windows. Nevertheless, malnutrition is a risk, particularly during fasting days with a very low-calorie restriction. For this reason, if you are a beginner, try to start by adopting a more permissive IF diet and with a longer eating window.

- **Dehydration** can become a problem, but it is easily circumvented. Various apps on the market can be installed on your phone to remind you to drink fluids regularly. Moreover, get into the habit of always having a bottle of water with you and setting yourself to finish it during the day.

- **Mood swings:** Remember that doing IF is your choice. During the first few days, it is normal to be irritable and angry with the whole world. What I can advise you is not to push yourself over the edge. If you realize that IF is not for you, no one forces you to continue. Mood swings, irregular bowel movements, and sleep disturbances may make you feel un-easy. These emotions should not be dismissed. If you are experiencing extreme discomfort while fasting, you should stop and consult your doctor.

~ CHAPTER 3 ~

THE RIGHT TYPE OF INTERMITTENT FASTING

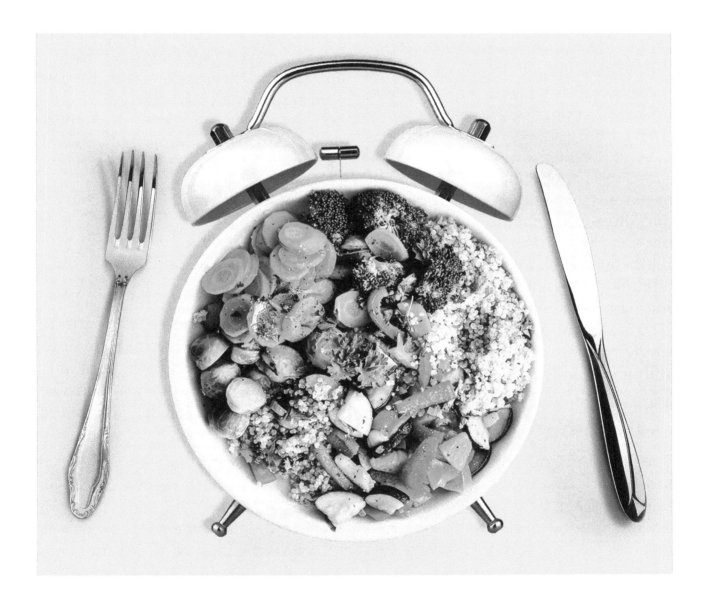

There are numerous Intermittent Fasting techniques, and choosing the most appropriate for your case is the first step towards success. This chapter will describe the various methods providing as much information as possible to guide you in an informed choice. However, during your journey, you may find that the chosen methodology is not the most suitable for you. For example, your body may not react adequately, or the diet may turn out to be too intense. Listening to your body is the most important thing; you are always in time to change your approach, and there is no shame in doing so. It doesn't always make sense to grit your teeth and evaluate how your body adapts to the new lifestyle. Especially for the most inexperienced, choosing a softer initial approach and a more forgiving diet is the best way to start with the right foot.

16:8 METHOD

The 16:8 method consists of limiting foods and calorie-containing beverages to a set time window of eight hours per day and abstaining from food for the remaining 16 hours.

This is probably the most popular fasting method; since the schedule is clear, it is hard to commit mistakes, if not intentionally. In addition, the 8-hour eating window can be decided in advance to adapt to your work and personal needs.

This cycle can be repeated as frequently as you like; I suggest starting just once or twice per week to give your body time to adapt to this method. Then, when you feel more confident, you can try a consecutive week or more, according to your needs.

The first thing to do to get started is picking your eight-hour window. The two most common choices are:

- **12 am to 8 pm**
- **9 am to 5 pm**

Put simply, if you decide to use the 12 am - 8 pm window, most of the Fasting will happen during the night, and the only real change to your lifestyle will be avoiding evening snacks and skipping breakfast.

Choosing instead the 9 am - 5 pm window, you can have a rich breakfast, lunch, and a light early dinner or snack in the late afternoon. However, you can experiment and pick the time frame that best fits your schedule.

For Intermittent Fasting to be effective, it is essential to maintain a balanced diet. This is not only valid for the 16:8 approach, but all the methods presented in this chapter.

It is important to balance each meal with a good variety of food:

- **Fruits:** Apples, bananas, berries, oranges, peaches, pears, etc.

- **Healthy fats:** Olive oil, avocados, and coconut oil

- **Sources of protein:** Meat, poultry, fish, legumes, eggs, nuts, seeds, etc.

- **Vegetables:** Broccoli, cauliflower, cucumbers, leafy greens, tomatoes, etc.

- **Whole grains:** Quinoa, rice, oats, barley, buckwheat, etc.

Also, I suggest avoiding drinking beverages that contain sugar or calories. Ideally, it would be best to stick to **water** only, but **unsweetened tea and coffee** are also okay.

16:8 intermittent fasting is probably the more straightforward method to follow and will help you save some money and time on cooking food each week. In addition, this method is not too stressful for the body and can be easily followed even for long periods.

The biggest drawback of this and other IF methods is overeating. As already said, during the eating window, some people could start to eat more than usual. This might lead to weight gain and digestive problems.

I suggest beginners start with the 16:8 approach and move into more challenging methods only when your body has fully adapted to this new lifestyle. In most cases, the 16:8 approach will already lead to excellent results.

14:10 METHOD

In some cases, starting with the 16:8 method is too complicated, or your body does not respond as you would expect to the diet. To avoid possible side effects caused by intermittent Fasting and relieve the pressure on your body, it is possible to switch to a 14:10 method.

This method is perfect for people who want to start gradually and is perfectly sustainable even for very long periods as it involves minimal changes to their lifestyle.

Unlike the 16:8 method, the eating window is longer (10 hours). This guarantees greater flexibility on managing meals and the possibility of having three meals a day without stringent time limits.

There are different eating windows that you could try; the most commons are:

- **7 am – 5 pm**
- **8 am – 7 pm**

There is enough time for a rich breakfast, a balanced lunch, and a light early dinner in both cases.

12:12 METHOD

The 12:12 approach is well-suited to beginners; some people even practice it without even knowing it. Following a 12-hour eating window is simple and does not require particular efforts; for example, one of the most commonly used windows is 8 am - 8 pm, which usually fits most people's schedules. By choosing this window, you will eat breakfast just after 8 am and finish dinner before 8 pm.

Unlike other intermittent fasting methods, this will cause minimal lifestyle changes for many people, and it is easily approachable by beginners who have never tried this type of diet.

12:12 is considered a very light diet with virtually no side effects. Obviously, it is always good to consult your doctor before starting a new diet, especially if you have pre-existing medical conditions. Compared to other, more intense diets, you can expect lower results. However, sticking to 12:12 could lead to overweight people losing 1 or 2 pounds a month.

You can consider this diet as one of the possible starting points to start your journey into Intermittent Fasting. Once your body gets used to this new lifestyle, it will be easier to restrict the eating window and apply slightly more challenging diets such as 16: 8 or 14:10.

20:4 METHOD

Stepping things up a notch from the 14:10 and 16:8 methods, the 20:4 method is a tough one to master, for it is rather unforgiving. People talk about this method of Intermittent Fasting as intense and highly restrictive. Still, they also say that the effects of living this method are almost unparalleled with all other tactics.

For the 20:4 method, you'll fast for 20 hours each day and squeeze all your meals, all your eating, and all your snacking into 4 hours. People who attempt 20:4 typically have two smaller meals or just one large meal and a few snacks during their 4-hour window to eat, and it is up to the individual which four hours of the day they devote to eating.

The trick for this method is to make sure you're not overeating or bingeing during that short eating window. It is all-too-easy to get hungry during the 20-hour fast and have that feeling then propel you into intense and unrealistic hunger or meal sizes after the fast period is over. So be careful if you try this method. If you're new to Intermittent Fasting, work your way up to this one gradually, and if you're working your way up already, only make the shift to 20:4 when you know you're ready. It would surely disappoint if all your progress with intermittent Fasting got hijacked by one poorly thought-out goal with the 20:4 method.

Furthermore, please consider that maintaining a 4-hour eating window for long periods is not recommended.

Having such a tight window is not only difficult for the body but also for your mind. It is essential to set our goals in advance and work in cycles. For example, you may decide to adopt 20: 4 initially for a week, evaluate the body's response, and then carry out a longer cycle if you feel fit to do so. The difficulties involved in this method should not be underestimated, and it is vital to listen to your body every step of the way.

I think this method is too aggressive for some types of people who, in my opinion, should avoid it; in these categories, we find:

- Pregnancy and breastfeeding women.

- Individuals under 18 years old.

- If you're underweight or have a history of an eating disorder.

- Athletes.

If you have a pre-existing medical condition such as insulin resistance or type 2 diabetes or you are taking medications, it is strongly recommended you consult your general practitioner before considering this method.

THE 5:2 DIET

The 5:2 diet is a calorie-limiting diet that follows a prescriptive program based on days of the week.

This method is particularly effective for very busy people who find it difficult to organize themselves with a fixed eating window during the week. The idea behind the 5: 2 diet is to normally eat for five days a week and drastically reduce the calories ingested for the remaining two days.

5: 2 can be considered a part-time diet that does not impose strict restrictions for most of the week, allowing us to eat chocolate, pasta, or any food we desire for five days. Obviously, to avoid nullifying the chances of success of this diet, the recommendation is to consume a normal number of calories during the week and avoid falling into the phenomenon of overeating.

During the two days of calorie restrictions, calorie intake should be limited to 500 calories for women and 600 for men. During the other five days, you should aim to consume around 2000 calories per day. This means that you are seeking to consume 3000 calories less or even more in an entire week.

Your 500-calorie days will help regulate hunger and insulin levels, naturally reducing your appetite, making it easier to meet the 2000 calorie limit for five days of the week.

No restrictions are imposed on the type of food we want to consume; the important thing is not to exceed the number of calories indicated. In terms of weight loss, following this diet strictly, a woman over 50 can expect to lose around 1lb per week. Of course, this figure can vary based on how physically active you are and how much you eat.

This diet method is not particularly intensive for the body, and for this reason, it can also be continued for long periods or until you reach the ideal weight.

If you feel that your goals are too ambitious, you can decide to do two or more cycles in order to insert some breaks between them so as not to make the diet too stressful. The duration of the breaks can vary; I personally recommend a week so as not to lose the healthy habits you have built.

Scheduling your meals during a 5:2 diet is not strictly required, but it might help achieve better results.

I suggest keeping your meals in 12 hours, between 7 am and 7 pm, avoiding late dinners. A more strict time window can be used if you look for faster results – i.e. from 7 am to 3 pm. By eating earlier in the day and extending the overnight fast, you will significantly help your metabolism.

For your 2000-calories days, you have the freedom to eat whatever you like; I have added to this book many healthy recipes that can help you organize your meal plan.

During your 500-calories days, you have to pay more attention to your diet, as it is very easy to reach and exceed 500 calories. Therefore, I suggest you focus on the following foods that usually guarantee a balanced calorie intake and allow you to create delicious recipes:

- Vegetables
- Fish
- Eggs
- Small portions of lean meat
- Soups

The easiest way to fit three meals into 500 calories is by eating a plant-based Mediterranean-style diet with plenty of fruits, vegetables, and legumes. Also, try to limit refined grains and avoid snacks during meals.

Regarding drinks, I would recommend you drink only water, but herbal tea and black coffee can be consumed if you want something different.

EAT STOP EAT

Brad Pilon invented the eat stop eat method while doing graduate research on short-term fasting at the University of Guelph. This method is straightforward and consists of fasting for 24 hours, twice a week, then eating "responsibly" for the other five days.

Eat stop eat falls in the group of methods associated with Intermittent Fasting dieting; unlike regular diets, calorie counting plays a secondary role with this method. Given the time restrictions, it becomes much more difficult to cheat and consume more calories than you should. Obviously, a minimum of willpower is required to respect the fasting periods and not overeat in the periods in which eating is allowed.

With *eat stop eat*, you can organize your week as you prefer; the important thing is to have two non-consecutive fasting days. This could be confusing at first, but you will always eat something on any calendar day when you adopt this method. For example, if you fast from 8 am on Tuesday to 8 am on Wednesday, you will try to have a meal just before 8 am on Tuesday and eat your next meal just after 8 am on Wednesday, fasting precisely 24 hours.

During fasting days, it is essential to maintain a high level of hydration. Therefore, especially if you decide to "eat stop eat" during hot periods, make an effort to drink frequently.

Like other Intermittent Fasting methods, *eat stop eat* acts on the metabolism; our body, when it is in a state of fasting for 12-36 hours, will begin to consume the glucose and then move on to burning fat. The state induced by Fasting is called *ketosis*. In this state, our body produces ketone from fat, using it as an energy source instead of carbohydrates. According to various researches, due to this temporary change in metabolism, intermittent Fasting can promote fat consumption in a much more effective way when compared to traditional diets.

Like all types of intermittent fasting diets also eat stop eat can have undesirable effects; among the most common we find:

- **Insufficient nutrient intake:** Some people may find it challenging to maintain a balanced diet during the five days of non-fasting. Not consuming enough calories at the correct times can make it very difficult to sustain the fasting period.

- **Low blood sugar:** Some people, especially those with diabetes, may find it difficult to maintain good blood sugar levels during fasting days. For this reason, it is not recommended to adopt this type of diet if you have medical conditions. Contact your doctor first.

- **Hormonal changes:** This type of diet can lead to changes in the production of metabolic and reproductive hormones. The effects caused by a change in hormone production are difficult to define due to the conflicting results found in the various papers published on the topic. At the moment, it is not easy to say whether these changes have a positive or negative impact on our bodies and which categories of individuals are affected.

- **Psychological impact:** Some research indicates that short-term Fasting may lead specific individuals to irritability, volatile moods, and reduced libido.

ALTERNATE DAY FASTING

Like most of the methods of Intermittent Fasting, this technique is straightforward to apply. On this diet, you fast every other day, but there are no restrictions on what you can eat on non-fasting days.

You can drink as much as you like during the fasting days, but you must limit yourself only to water, unsweetened coffee, and unsweetened tea. Any other type of drink should be avoided so as not to compromise the diet. Moreover, during the fasting days, it is allowed to consume about 500 calories.

If this approach sounds similar to the 5: 2 method, you are right; you can consider alternate day fasting as a more challenging version of the 5: 2 method.

When and how you decide to consume your calories allowance does not affect the results obtained.

Various studies have been conducted on this, and the division of calories between breakfast, lunch, and dinner does not seem to impact the final result. Therefore, this method may be more suitable for some people who, due to their multiple commitments, find it challenging to manage strict time constraints in their diet since you can freely decide how and when to consume the calories of the day.

We reduce calories to 500 on fasting days instead of completely zeroing them out to be able to sustain this type of diet for more extended periods. Consuming zero calories could bring more significant benefits in terms of weight loss and body purification in the short term but have adverse effects on our body during a prolonged diet.

In terms of weight loss, following this method, you can expect a loss of between 3% and 8% of your body weight over a period of 2 to 12 weeks. The reason for all this variance in results lies in the boundary conditions. For example, an obese and physically active person will tend to lose much more than a slightly overweight person who does not engage in physical activity.

As I said before, you can structure your fasting days as you like in terms of calorie breakdown and what to eat during meals. In my experience, I have seen people handling better fasting days using one of the following approaches:

- One "big" meal in the late afternoon to consume all 500 calories.

- One "big" meal at lunchtime to consume all 500 calories.

- Two small meals, one around 11 am and one around 5 pm.

At the end of this book, I've added plenty of recipes that might be suitable for your dieting needs, but to give you an idea of what you can consume during your fasting days, here is a shortlist of ideas:

- Eggs and vegetables

- Yogurt with berries

- Grilled fish or lean meat with vegetables

- Soup and a piece of fruit

- Salad with lean meat

Alternate day fasting is perfect for losing weight for most people, but if you suffer from any congenital disease, I recommend contacting your doctor. In addition, it has been proven that alternate day fasting can cause some existing conditions to worsen, such as Gilbert syndrome.

SPONTANEOUS MEAL SKIPPING

Spontaneous meal skipping is, by far, the easiest method of intermittent Fasting; many people do it without even realizing it. For example, do you remember when you were teenagers and skipped a meal because you wake up too late on the weekend? Spontaneous meal skipping is practically skipping a meal every now and then when you get the chance.

This method is ideal, especially for beginners who are approaching intermittent Fasting for the first time. My advice is to start by skipping a couple of meals a week and eventually increase to three or four. During this process, it is essential to pay attention to our body; spontaneous meal skipping is one of the IF methods with fewer side effects, but the risk of feeling tired or edgy exists. The best ways to avoid any side effects are to focus on a healthy and balanced diet and avoid skipping meals that are too close together. For example, I strongly advise against skipping two consecutive meals when using this method.

Compared to the other types of IF exposed in this book, the results you can get with this method are less impressive; you can expect to lose around 1 or 2 pounds per month. Nonetheless, you can consider this method as your gateway to the world of Intermittent Fasting and a first step into changing your lifestyle and reducing your weekly calories intake.

∽CHAPTER 4∾
LET'S BEGIN!

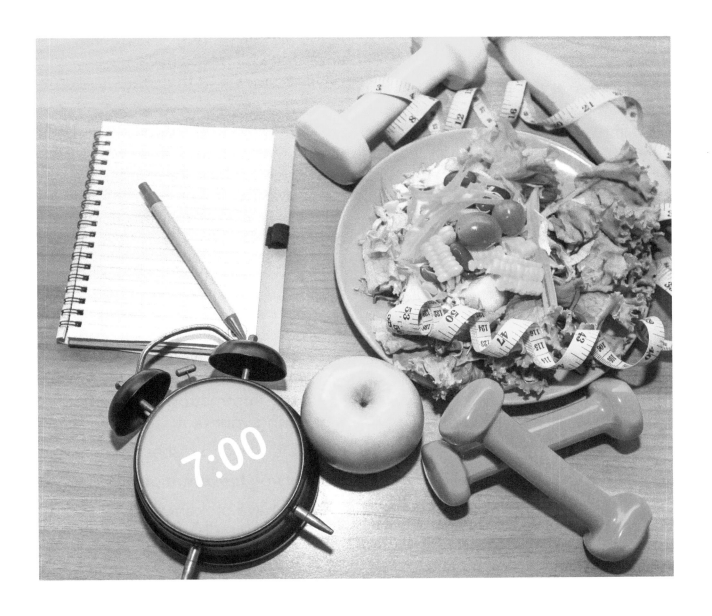

HOW DO YOU START YOUR INTERMITTENT FASTING?

In the previous chapter, I did my best to explain the various intermittent fasting methods to give you an idea of the basic principles of this diet. This chapter will detail how to organize an intermittent fasting diet that leads you to the desired results.

First, I advise you to take an empty notebook that will become your diet diary.

It is essential to create the habit of recording all critical information in this notebook daily; this will allow you to analyze how your diet is progressing and if any changes to the chosen approach are necessary.

The first thing to write in your notebook is your goal. Think carefully about what you want to get from this diet and write it down. Think of this front page as a contract with yourself that binds you to achieve your goal.

Next, suppose you have decided to use a variant of the IF diet that is not spontaneous meal skipping. In that case, I recommend that you write down a sort of calendar in your notebook that clearly defines the time slots or days in which you have to fast or reduce your calorie intake.

Depending on the duration of the diet, you might have to review this calendar multiple times. I suggest making a habit of checking it on the first of each month. Do not think of this calendar as immutable; especially if you are inexperienced, you may realize that you have chosen the wrong days or times and that they do not fit your lifestyle.

If you feel the need, you can go back to examine your calendar and modify it when more appropriate; the important thing is to make an effort to follow it and not give up at the first difficulty.

As a third step, we want to create the habit of recording daily information in your notebook about how the diet is progressing. Of course, you can decide to write whatever you want in your notebook, but I believe the following information is essential for monitoring your diet:

- Mealtimes and dishes consumed.
- How you feel emotionally.
- If you have broken your diet for any reason, describe how and when.

Recording this information will help you to identify patterns later; here are some examples:

- You may realize that the time of one or more of your meals tends to be at the limit of the fasting window, and reconsider the window chosen

- You may notice that your mood worsens on a particular day of the week, and if you are applying the 5: 2 method, you may want to reconsider the allocation of fasting days.

- You may notice that you tend to stop dieting too often to get results and decide to change methodology.

- Etc.

By keeping a journal, what you might discover depends on the accuracy of the information recorded and how critical you are with yourself. Some people find it very useful, while others tend to stop using it after a few weeks. This method may or may not suit you, but I advise you to give it a chance before discarding it a priori.

TIPS AND TRICKS FOR A SUCCESSFUL DIET

How many times did you happen to start with a diet and then fail to complete it? How many times did you decide that it was time to lose weight and then give up after a few tiring weeks of dieting?

If I think back to my youth and all the diets I tried, my answer is "many!" and we are probably in the same boat. The truth is, starting a diet is easy; getting it to completion is damn hard, but you probably know better than me.

In this section, I want to reveal some tricks that I have collected over the years of working with various clients. I hope that the tips contained here will help you to be able to follow a diet from start to finish in the best possible way.

SET YOUR SMART GOALS

Every person loses weight for a specific reason. Your ultimate goal could be to lose that belly that makes you feel uncomfortable, or you are aiming for a more drastic transformation, but whatever your ultimate goal, it is essential to set a series of intermediate goals. These goals must be clear, evaluable, achievable, and it is for this reason, they are defined as SMART. **SMART** is an acronym that defines the main characteristics that one of your intermediate goals should have:

- **Specific:** You should be specific with your goals and how you plan to meet them.

- **Measurable:** You need to be able to measure your goals so that you can understand the progress

- **Attainable:** You should only choose goals that are reasonable and can be achieved.

- **Relevant:** Choose goals that are truly important to you and that you care about.

- **Timely/time-bound:** It is essential to give yourself time to reach a specific goal to create the psychological urge to achieve it.

An example of a SMART goal could be: "I want to be able to get into that old pair of jeans that I love so much by the end of February." A goal of this type is measurable since we are talking about losing weight to a specific size, it has a deadline, it is something I care about, and it does not seem like a utopia.

In my experience, I would recommend that you choose a small SMART goal each month. This will allow you to always focus on your diet and help you keep the right trajectory to reach the final goal.

REWARD YOURSELF

For each goal, you can decide on a different reward that is unlocked only when that goal is reached

Okay, let's say you've achieved one of your SMART goals; it's time to enjoy your reward!

Here are some ideas:

- **Book a nice massage:** In addition to relaxing and enjoying a bit of tranquility, a good massage can improve blood circulation and improve mood.

- **Go to a hike:** Why not organize a hike and go for beautiful walks in the middle of a lovely green area? It will help you to improve your fitness and at the same time get away from the daily routine.

- **A new cookbook:** This could be an opportunity to discover new cuisines or find new ideas for delicious dishes. For example, have you ever considered buying a **Sous Vide**? It is a perfect tool to keep the food's nutritional properties unaltered and discover new flavors.

- **A bike:** Why not get a new bike? It will help you create healthy habits and discover new places alone or with the people you love.

- **A vacation:** For your ultimate goal, you could treat yourself to an unforgettable holiday where you can show off your newfound physical shape!

- **A new blender:** It can be helpful to prepare healthy meals and smoothies.

- **Aromatherapy Oils:** Sleeping is one of the most critical phases of the day for anyone trying to lose weight. Aromatherapy is exceptional for relaxing the body and improve sleep quality. You may decide to reward yourself by purchasing a set of essential oils; the best to help you sleep are lavender camomile and jasmine but feel free to try what you like most.

DEAL WITH HUNGER PANGS

It is customary to suffer from hunger pangs by doing any diet, and it is essential to know how to manage them. If you, too, like many, suffer from hunger pangs, the tricks listed below could help you stay true to your diet plan:

- **Eat breakfast:** It might sound like a trivial piece of advice, but breakfast is the most important meal of the day. If the style of intermittent Fasting you have chosen allows it, try not to skip breakfast.

- **Stay hydrated:** According to Dr. Melinda Jampolis, you should drink at least eight glasses of water a day. Also, keep in mind that sometimes what you think is hunger pangs are a sign of inadequate hydration.

- **Spice up your meals:** According to Dr. Alan Hirsch of the Chicago Smells and Taste Treatment and Research Fundations, adding spice to your meals can help fool your brain and inhibit hunger.

- **Exercise regularly:** It might seem counterintuitive, but according to a study published in 2008 by the American Journal of Physiology, any form of exercise helps regulate appetite and control hunger pangs.

- **Eat slowly:** This falls into the "grandmother's advice" category, but it was recently proven by a study conducted by the University of Rhodes that eating slowly helps convey a sense of fullness.

- **Chew gum:** Eating low-calorie gum before and after eating can help reduce hunger symptoms and consume fewer calories.

- **Stay busy:** Have you ever tried to have a busy day at work that you only realize in the late afternoon that you haven't even had lunch? Keeping our mind busy helps to ignore hunger pangs; during fasting times, try to keep yourself busy with activities that engage your mind.

KNOW WHAT TO EAT AND PRACTICE PORTION CONTROL

Eating the right foods during an intermittent fasting diet is as crucial as fasting during the correct periods. For this reason, in this book, I have included many recipes that can help you plan your meals and be a source of inspiration for your meal plan. Also, if you are interested in eating healthy foods that keep their nutritional properties intact, I would recommend buying a **Sous Vide**.

Sous Vide is a French culinary technique that allows you to cook food at a precise temperature in a water bath. As a result, your food will turn out perfectly every time, without ever burning or overcooking. This technique is perfect for cooking every cut of meat or fish; from the most tender to some tough cuts, the result will always be excellent. Sous Vide is also great for cooking vegetables at a precise temperature, preventing them from getting mushy and losing their taste, or it can be used to prepare amazing desserts. I started using this technique a few years ago, and I was pleasantly surprised.

I chose not to add recipes for the *Sous Vide* in this book since it is not a kitchen utensil that everyone has at home but, if you are interested, I would like to suggest this recipe book, *"Sous Vide Cookbook: 600 Easy Foolproof Recipes to Cook Meat, Seafood, and Vegetables in Low Temperature for Everyone, from Beginner to Ad-*

vanced" by *Sophia Marchesi*. It is relatively inexpensive, and it has over 600 detailed recipes with complete nutritional values.

Intermittent Fasting is a type of diet that allows you to eat what you want as long as you do so during the permitted periods of the day. However, this does not mean that you are allowed to eat without restraint; it is essential to limit portions when possible and not eat more than necessary.

When it comes to portion control, there are a few tips that you could find helpful:

- **Use a smaller plate:** It might sound silly, but you can trick your brain into thinking you have eaten more if you use smaller plates.

- **Only one carbohydrate source at a time:** When you plan your meals, consider using only one source of carbohydrates per meal to limit your intake.

- **Measuring cups can be your best friend:** If you have difficulty measuring the right quantities of food, you can use measuring cups to avoid errors and consume only what you need.

- **20-minute rule:** If you think you are still hungry after finishing a meal, wait 20 minutes to allow the sense of satiety to reach the brain. If after 20 minutes you are still hungry, then you haven't eaten enough.

- **Ask for less:** There is no shame in asking for smaller portions when eating out.

BE PATIENT

One of the most frequent reasons why a diet fails is impatience, and Intermittent Fasting is no different from other diets in this aspect. To see the first results, any diet requires a certain amount of time, which can vary from person to person.

Usually, Intermittent Fasting takes at least ten days for you to start seeing the first changes, but it will take at least two weeks to see the first significant weight reduction.

During the first ten days, you will begin to feel less bloated, but the scale will hardly show any noticeable changes; nevertheless, you will feel better with your body and begin to see yourself thinner in the mirror. During the second week of the diet, people usually start to lose the first few pounds, and the change will become more noticeable.

What I've given you is just an average estimation, and I do not want to deceive you; various factors influence how quickly your body can lose weight. On some of them, such as nutrition and physical activity, you have complete control, while on other factors, unfortunately, you do not.

We must take into account that our body is no longer twenty years old, and for this reason, the results may be delayed. However, given my experience with multiple clients of various ages and builds, I can tell you that **a person who follows Intermittent Fasting regularly should see the first results no later than four weeks.**

BREAKING YOUR FAST

No one is perfect, and we all know that it is challenging to follow a diet on certain days. Being tempted to break the fast is very common and has happened to everyone at least once. If we decide to break the fast when we shouldn't, the important thing is "to limit the damage as much

as possible." In this short paragraph, I will provide suggestions that may be trivial for some of you but are still good to remember.

- **Choose foods high in nutrients:** Plan out how you will prepare or obtain a nutrient-dense meal that fits your diet plan. If you are out and about or just really hungry when you are breaking your fast, for example, you may want to eat a small snack until you can eat your scheduled meal. Healthy smoothies or soups, such as a Green Smoothie with Apple, Avocado, and Spinach or Spicy Cauliflower Soup, are excellent choices because they are high in nutrients and fiber. They will also help you avoid overeating by filling your stomach. A tablespoon of coconut oil, MCT (Medium-Chain Triglycerides) oil, or another healthy fat is another choice.

- **Avoid empty calories, refined carbohydrates, and ultra-processed foods**, as they will not provide your body with the nourishing nutrients it requires after a fast. If you want your body to rebuild stronger during the growing phase, avoid foods that provide damaged building blocks, such as trans fats and inflammation-inducing vegetable oils. Cakes, cookies, white bread, pasta, pies, processed foods, sugary drinks, diet sodas, vegetable oil sources, and margarine should all be replaced with real whole foods and natural drinks that fit your diet.

- **Avoid consuming alcoholic beverages:** When breaking a fast, it's not a good idea to drink booze. If you choose to drink alcohol before your first meal, keep in mind that it will intensify the effects, so wait until after you've eaten or paired it with food.

PICK THE RIGHT DRINK!

In some cases, the drinks make the difference between the success and failure of a diet. For example, some may think that beer, a glass of wine, or a soft drink can't do any harm, but constantly choosing to drink the wrong products could sabotage the weight loss process.

For this reason, it is advisable to avoid as much as possible drinks that are not on this list:

- **Water:** The best choice!
- **Tea:** If you enjoy tea, you'll be pleased to learn that this hot beverage goes hand in hand with the goal of Intermittent Fasting. Tea also aids in the reduction of hunger. Avoid any sugar.
- **Coffee:** Contains caffeine, which boosts alertness and aids in weight loss. Caffeine, on the other hand, increases metabolism and aids weight loss. As a result, drinking coffee while Fasting is a great way to control hunger and burn more fat. Avoid any sugar.
- **Apple Cider Vinegar:** Most apple cider vinegar comprises water and acids like acetic acid and malic acid. Appropriately three calories are contained in 15 ml (one tablespoon) of apple cider vinegar. Ideal for weight loss!

KNOW YOUR BMI AND HOW TO CALCULATE IT

Before starting any type of diet, it is essential to know your status and how much overweight you are; an easy way to do this is to calculate the *Body Mass Index (BMI)*.

The BMI is a measure that uses your height and weight to work out if your weight is healthy. The BMI calculation divides an adult's weight (in kilograms) by height (in meters) squared. This index is a great way to track weight fluctuations, and I suggest recording the variations daily.

It is essential always to weigh yourself under the same conditions; for example, if you decide to weigh yourself in the morning on an empty stomach after a shower, try always to keep this approach.

Various online BMI calculators can help you, especially if you don't feel like spending time on stones/pounds/kilograms conversions; here are some helpful links:

https://patient.info/doctor/bmi-calculator-calculator

https://www.calculator.net/bmi-calculator.html

https://www.nhlbi.nih.gov/health/educational/lose_wt/BMI/bmicalc.htm

In case you want to calculate your BMI manually, or you are just curious to understand the logic applied, you can use one of these examples as a reference to calculate yours.

How to check BMI (Imperial Units)

Formula: weight (lbs) x 703 / height (squared inches)

Example: If you weigh 150lbs and your height is 65 (5'5"), then you will compute your BMI as:

150/(65 x 65) x 703 = 24.96

How to check BMI (Metric Units)

Formula: weight (kg) / height (metres squared)

Example: If you weigh 68kg and your height is 1.65m, then you will compute your BMI as:

68/(1.65 x 1.65) = 24.98

Left out of context, the BMI is just a number without much use, but you can refer to the following table to understand in which category you are and how the Intermittent Fasting diet affects your weight.

CATEGORY	BMI
Underweight	Below 18.5
Healthy weight	18.5 – 24.9
Overweight	25.0 – 29.9
Obese	30.0 and higher

Keep in mind that weight fluctuations will not always be downwards. For example, if you measure your BMI every day, on some days it is totally natural that your BMI may increase. This could be due to several reasons:

- Eating more than you should the previous day.
- You haven't emptied your bowels in the morning yet.
- Slightly inaccurate measurements can always happen.
- Etc…

I suggest not focusing on the result of the single day but looking at the trend of the week or the month to understand if you are aligned with your weight loss goals or if you need to consider corrections to your diet or your lifestyle. Then, try to record this data as accurately as possible in your diet diary so that you have as much information as possible at your disposal in case you want to make any changes.

I once asked my "finance consultant husband" if he knew anything about macros, and he told me that he uses them all the time to automate tasks in Microsoft Excel. You will be happy to know that in the context of diets and Intermittent Fasting, Excel and spreadsheets are not involved! "Macro" is short for macronutrients, the three main categories of nutrients (proteins, carbohydrates, and fats) that make up our diet. So basically, when a person counts their macros, they measure the grams of these nutrients they are getting. Therefore, keeping track of macros is nothing incredibly complex and consists of keeping track of what we eat in a journal or an app to know how to quantify our daily consumption of the three main categories of nutrients.

If you are looking for Apps designed to track your macros, there are plenty of options on the market. Here are some that I've tried with my clients:

- MyFitnessPal

- Lose It!

- My Macros+

Also, several of these apps feature a barcode scanner that you can use to retrieve the nutrients of every product you are cooking automatically; this will make it easier to understand your daily macros.

Let's take a step back now, and before starting to talk about how to measure macros and set daily goals, let's try to understand what these nutrients are in detail.

Carbohydrates: This category includes sugars, starches, and fibers. Carbohydrates are broken down into glucose to immediately provide energy to the body or glycogen to be stored in the liver and muscles. Carbohydrates provide an average of 4 calories per gram and usually represent the dominant part of the calories a person consumes in a day. There is an endless debate about whether carbohydrates are more or less good, and experts still disagree about it.

Still, many studies currently suggest getting between 45% and 65% of your daily calories from carbohydrates.

Fats: Among the three main macronutrients, fats have the most calories per gram (9). Fat consumption is essential to support body functions such as producing hormones, absorbing nutrients, and regulating body temperature. There are various high-fat diets, but it is generally suggested to gain between 20% and 35% of your daily calories from this nutrient. Examples of high-fat foods are butter, avocado, meat, and fatty fish.

Proteins: Proteins are essential to support functions such as building tissues and producing hormones and enzymes. Like carbohydrates, one gram of protein provides 4 calories. Therefore, obtaining between 10% and 35% of our daily calories from protein foods is advisable. Some examples of protein-rich foods are fish, lentils, and chicken.

Now that you know what macronutrients are and what they are for, let's understand how many we need per day to maintain a healthy lifestyle. The simplest way to understand the ideal quantity is to apply the following formula:

10 x weight (kg) + 6.25 x height (cm) – 5 x age (years) – 161

Also, the result has to be multiplied by a coefficient based on your lifestyle:

- **Sedentary:** x1.2 - Almost no exercise.

- **Lightly active:** x1.375 - Some light exercise, less than three days a week.

- **Moderately active:** x1.55 - Moderate exercise at least three days a week.

- **Very active:** x1.725 - Intensive exercise every day.

- **Extra active:** x1.9 - Intensive exercise two or more times per day.

Some of you may be confused about calculating your macros or simply not used to using the metric system but don't worry; various online calculators can help us. For instance, this website is excellent to get the numbers you are looking for:

https://www.calculator.net/macro-calculator.html.

Once you have your macros, tracking them is pretty simple. First, decide on your ideal macronutrients breakdown. A classic approach to achieve your daily macros goals can be:

- **Carbs:** 45–65% of total calories.

- **Fats:** 20–35% of total calories.

- **Proteins:** 10–35% of total calories.

To keep track of the number of proteins, fats and carbohydrates ingested, you can create a meal plan using the recipes with nutritional values contained in this book or, as already mentioned above, rely on Apps. By scanning the barcodes of the products, these Apps can record the nutritional values of every single ingredient and guide you in building your meal plan.

DIRTY FAST VS CLEAN FAST

You may not be aware of it or have only heard the term a few times, but there are two types of Fasting called "dirty" and "clean" derived from two different schools of thought.

Clean and dirty fasting are terms that refer to what breaks a fast; for some dieticians, only water should be consumed during a fasting period, while for others, low-calorie drinks are allowed, such as stevia and MCT oil.

We follow a clean fasting approach if we strictly follow an intermittent fasting method and drink only water or non-caloric beverages such as coffee and black tea during fasting periods. If we follow the clean strategy during fasting periods, it is essential to stay hydrated by consuming a lot of water. It is also crucial to avoid adding lemon slices, herbs, or flavorings that introduce undesired calories.

The dirty fasting approach is much more permissive and allows you to consume food or drinks during fasting periods as long as they have less than 50 calories. However, it is essential to note that this type of fasting, although easier to manage, will produce worse results in terms of weight loss than clean fasting. Furthermore, using dirty Fasting exposes you to the risk of mistakenly ingesting more than the allowable calories, potentially nullifying some of your sacrifices.

During the dirty fasting window, there are different food and beverages that you can consume; here are some ideas if you decide to try this approach:

- 1 tbsp maple syrup
  (17 calories, 14g carbs)
- 1 tsp MCT oil
  (38 calories, 0g carbs) x 100% fat
- 1 tbsp cream
  (30 calories, 0.5g carbs)
- 1 tbsp 2% cow's milk
  (18 calories, 1g of carbs)
- 2 tbsp almond milk (10 calories, 1g carbs)
- 1 tsp honey
  (20 calories, 6g carbs)
- Water + juice of 1 lemon
  (14 calories, 0g carbs)
- 1 tbsp aspartame
  (35 calories, 7g carbs)
- 1 cup bone broth
  (40 calories, 3g carbs)
- Sugar-free chewing gum
  (0 calories, 0g carbs)
- Stevia
  (0 calories, 0g carbs)
- Splenda/sucralose
  (0 calories, 0g carbs)

Choosing whether to adopt a clean or dirty fasting window is a personal choice dictated by the needs of the individual and your tolerance to fasting. If you are new to the world of Intermittent Fasting, you may want to start with a simple diet like 14:10 and a dirty fasting window and then progress to more intensive diets based on your goals and your body's reactions. Both methods lead to results and are legitimate, but greater sacrifice is often associated with better results. Having said that, I invite you not to be in a hurry on your weight loss path and choose the method that best suits your level of experience.

THE MINDSET IS EVERYTHING

Losing weight is about more than just diet and exercise; everything starts from the right mindset. Applying a diet is easy in theory, but if it were easy in practice, everyone would lose weight without the slightest effort, and it would not make sense for me to write books about this topic. Unfortunately, in practice, many of the most renowned and "bullet-proof" diets fail because those who put them into practice do not have the correct mindset, and Intermittent Fasting is no exception.

"Shifting your mindset about how to lose weight is the biggest factor in losing weight," says Kathryn Smerling, a therapist based in New York City. *"We can't shift our weight from the outside without realizing the correct inner resolve and intention."*

Working on a person's mindset requires a lot of time, effort, and sometimes the support of experienced professionals in the sector. In this chapter, I do not set myself the goal of changing your mindset overnight, but I want to give you, in my small way, some advice that I hope can help you reach your weight loss goals.

The first thing you must avoid when starting a diet is having the thought "I want to fix myself" in your head or, even worse, being disgusted by your physical appearance highlighting all your flaws in your mind. This approach is highly destructive and leads many people to embark on extreme diets beyond their abilities and then quit a few days or weeks later, generating a negative state of frustration.

To reinforce the concept that you have to change your mindset to approach a new diet in a positive way, there is research by the University of Syracuse that links being dissatisfied with your body to mental resistance to physical changes even simply thinking that you are overweight leads to further weight gain, according to 2015 research published in the International Journal of Obesity.

At the base of this, there is the theory that it is our mind, first of all, to define us. So, for example, a person who perceives himself in shape will tend to be more confident and will create the ideal environment for this person to train and further improve. But, unfortunately, the reverse is also true, and a person who is unsure of her appearance will create a hostile environment around her where it is more difficult to achieve even reasonable goals.

Fortunately, our mind is a uniquely flexible tool that can be trained to improve our perception and reduce the negativity we create around us. In this chapter, I do not set myself the goal of taking the place of industry experts, but I want to share with you a series of tips that I hope will help you take the first steps to improve your mindset.

START ALWAYS FROM YOUR WHY

First, you must identify why you want to embark on a journey that will change your body.

Second, you must be honest with yourself to determine the reason that pushes you to change.

For example, in my case, it took me a while to accept that what initially pushed me to diet years ago was the teasing of my classmates. I found myself having to acknowledge my weakness against the pressure exerted by other people until I realized that my wanting to lose weight was not for them but for myself. It took me a while to admit that I felt trapped in a body not mine and that I wanted to free my true self. I recommend to all my clients to spend some time on this point. Don't be in a rush to start your diet; take a few days to think first and be sure to find the right motivations. Remember that there is always time to start a diet and consider this as the preparatory work you are doing to ensure its success.

EVERY DECISION YOU TAKE IS IMPORTANT

Your relationship with food could lead you to make bad decisions.

During a diet, temptations come in various forms, and we are constantly under scrutiny. Our choices ultimately determine the success of a diet, and a wrong decision can lead to another, creating a chain effect that will lead to abandoning our initial plans. It is not easy to avoid this but what you can do is write.

Writing how you feel about your food choices will help you create a connection between your thoughts and decisions and help you understand why you have chosen less healthy food in certain situations.

SMART GOALS

We have already talked about smart goals, and I will not elaborate further. These goals can help you shift your focus to what you have control over and work towards achievable and meaningful goals. This will create a state of gratification that will propel you towards the next goal.

SURROUND YOURSELF WITH POSITIVE PEOPLE

Many people dislike change, dislike seeing others succeed, and tend to be destructive and judge others. These people are a threat to our success and must be eliminated from our lives.

Surround yourself with positive people who support you and want to see you succeed. Difficult moments in a journey of this type will always happen and having people around you who have the power to make you feel better can make the difference.

TAKE A BREATH

I recommend that you create a habit of taking a few minutes at the beginning of the day to slow down and simply focus on the act of breathing. This will help you connect with your body and focus on your goals and what is really important to you.

I have found this breathing technique very useful in the past: lie on your back with your legs extended and place one hand on your stomach and one on your chest. Breathe in through your nose for four seconds, hold for two and then exhale through your mouth for six. With each breath, the hand placed on your stomach should be the only one to rise or fall. Repeat until you feel focused and ready to start your day.

ALL-OR-NOTHING THINKING IS DANGEROUS

"Only a Sith deals in absolutes" it's one of my favorite Star Wars quotes. When many people embark on a diet, they tend to set absurd and unrealistic goals in a rush to get results. The most predictable result is to start failing to achieve any intermediate results and start thinking that there is no point in continuing the diet and that it is all a failure.

One of the most important pieces of advice I can give you is to abandon the "all-or-nothing" mentality immediately. Instead, you have to focus on actually achievable goals and understand that failing some intermediate goals during a diet is fine. Especially if you are a beginner, you will find it difficult initially to set realistic goals, and there will always be a certain probability of "failure."

As you gain experience and learn about your body, you will begin to choose more achievable goals reducing the chance of "failure."

I find talking about failure not correct. In my opinion, you can see every diet as a journey, and not reaching an intermediate goal within the established time frame is not a failure in itself. Instead, it is crucial to objectively evaluate the improvements obtained not only from a physical point of view but also from a mental one. So, for example, if you have not lost the weight you had set for yourself after a month, but you still feel more fit, toned, and happy, it makes no sense to consider this a failure just because you didn't reach your intermediate goal. Your path will simply be different from your expectations.

DON'T BE HARD ON YOURSELF

It is no mystery that many people tend to judge themselves more severely than they would with another person. Unfortunately, being hard on oneself is a behavior that is often inherent in our being and is terribly difficult to correct. Try to voice your internal monologue, and instead of judging yourself severely, try to apply the same yardstick you would use for a dear friend. Your behavior will not change overnight, but I can assure you that your way of thinking will start to change after a few weeks.

STOP CLASSIFYING FOOD AS GOOD OR BAD

Making a diet based on hamburgers and fries is not feasible, but at the same time imposing strict food categorizations can be harmful in adopting a new lifestyle for an extended period. Occasionally you will be tempted to eat a cookie or drink a glass of wine more than you should, and sometimes you will succumb to these temptations. If, from the point of view of the diet, this is not recommended, at the same time it is essential to understand that sometimes our body and our mind need something more.

Sometimes breaking the rules in a diet is normal and should not be experienced as right or wrong in absolute terms. For example, if you ate that extra cookie, you probably needed it, and you don't have to feel guilty. The important thing is that you know that this is an exception and does not become the norm.

CHEAT MEALS

Let's face it, following a diet all the time without ever falling into temptation is practically impossible; even the most mentally strong and focused on the ultimate goal will sooner or later take a slight misstep. Unfortunately, there is no way to reduce to zero the mistakes we might make while on a diet; the foods we most desire are temptations that are there, waiting for a single moment of weakness.

What I always suggest to my clients is not to block these temptations but to channel them into the very structure of the diet. The basic idea is that if we cannot effectively combat these temptations, we can at least try to regulate them not to destroy the results obtained and avoid the inevitable sense of guilt that afflicts us immediately after consuming what we desired.

The sense of guilt is our most dangerous enemy. When we have been following a diet for days or weeks, eating a dessert or having a drink usually gives us an immediate sense of satisfaction, followed by a sense of guilt and failure. These feelings are dangerous and could undermine our self-confidence and ability to complete the diet. By incorporating some "cheat meals" into our schedule, we can avoid these negative feelings and instead consider these meals as rewards for following the diet in the best way.

How often you want to have these cheat meals is up to you. However, I suggest that my clients who are approaching Intermittent Fasting starting with one cheat meal a week. As we have previously seen, there are variants of Intermittent Fasting that are not particularly strict on what we eat but, obviously, recommend a reasonable consumption of calories. In many cases eating a cheat meal once every two weeks is more than enough since the restrictions applied by this type of diet are mainly on the fasting window and not on what we eat. If you have decided to adopt a more restrictive portion control with macro tracking, having a cheat meal a week may be necessary to be able to follow the diet in the long term.

The most important thing, as already said, is to avoid the sense of guilt and failure that could lead you to abandon your goals. If you need more incentives to continue the diet, choose a higher frequency of cheat meals and slowly reduce it. Remember that dieting is not about spending two months of hell every year; it is about maintaining a sustainable lifestyle with the right balance between sacrifices and results.

EXERCISING WHILE FASTING

The key to losing weight is not only fasting but also physical activity. Exercising while following an Intermittent Fasting diet is not dangerous, but some precautions must be taken. For example, some people argue that exercising in a fasted state can lead to muscle loss, but in reality, this risk is minimal if not non-existent for classic intermittent fasting diets.

Diet and exercise instead create a perfect synergy, accelerating weight loss and improving fitness more quickly.

In this book, it is not my intention to play the role of a personal trainer as there are people far more experienced than me in the field. Still, I would like to share with you a series of tips that I am sure will help you get the best from the combination of diet and physical exercise.

WHEN TO WORKOUT DURING INTERMITTENT FASTING

Usually, the best time to do a workout when you practice Intermittent

Fasting is as soon as you wake up. You should avoid training or eating too late in the evening as this could alter deep and REM sleep levels and, consequently, sleep quality.

Some types of training can be carried out on an empty stomach, while for others, it is advisable to eat a meal (ideally a light one) to have enough energy to carry out the workout effectively. If you plan to perform a high-intensity workout it is advisable to have at least a light snack. Personally, I would not be able to do even a HIIT circuit after 10+ hours of fasting. This is obviously subjective, and some people are better off training on an empty stomach; as always, I invite you to listen to your body and try what works best for you.

CHOSE THE TYPE OF WORKOUT BASED ON YOUR MACROS

It is also important to organize your workouts so that you do not eat immediately afterward. Various studies show that waiting two to three hours before eating after a workout helps to increase growth hormone levels, increasing the rate at which fat is burned.

This rule does not apply to everything; there are situations in which it is advisable to wait a shorter period before consuming a meal; for example, if you have done high-intensity training.

Also, it is advisable to wait only half an hour and take carbohydrates and about 20g of protein for strength training. In principle, if you have done a strength workout, you will need to consume more carbohydrates that day. In contrast, exercises such as cardio and HIIT (High-Intensity Interval Training) can be done in one day with lower carbohydrate consumption.

CONSIDER THE TYPE OF FAST

One of the elements to choose the type of training is to consider what intermittent fasting diet you are doing. For example, if you are on an extreme diet like 20: 4, it is advisable to limit yourself to low-intensity training such as yoga, pilates, and walking. On the other hand, if you follow a less aggressive diet with a reduced fasting window, you can introduce HIIT, weight lifting, and more intense types of training.

CARDIO

Cardio is a perfect activity during Intermittent Fasting. In addition to preventing the risk of stroke and heart disease, it promotes weight loss. However, it is essential to note that being in a fasted state, your performance will tend to decline and will be as good as your body has adapted to consuming fat instead of sugar for energy. Therefore, if you decide to do some cardio activity, I suggest you eat immediately after the workout and not wait the two or three hours previously suggested. Reintegrating energy after this type of activity is essential, and in this case, delaying the post-workout meal would not bring any kind of advantage.

Examples of cardio exercises you could try are:

- Jumping rope
- Jogging
- Swimming
- Cycling
- Water aerobics
- Dancing
- Rowing
- Martial arts
- Hiking
- Volleyball
- Basketball
- Soccer
- Racquetball

HIIT

HIIT is based on cycles of intense activity with minimal rest phases. As the name suggests, it is a type of intense training that should be avoided if you are on a demanding intermittent fasting diet. This type of training is incredible to increase the levels of HGH (Human Growth Hormone), favor the consumption of fat reserves, and increase stamina.

WEIGHT LIFTING

Combining weight lifting with intermittent Fasting is legitimate and can lead to great results if done correctly. The important thing is that you keep in mind the state in which you are going to train. When you train during a fasting window, likely, your glycogen stores have already been used up, and as weightlifting is a stressful type of training for the body, eating a meal immediately after a workout is essential. For this reason, you may want to organize your weight lifting sessions so that they take place after your meals.

YOGA AND INTERMITTENT FASTING

I decided to write a separate section on Yoga because it is one of the best physical activities to do during an Intermittent Fasting diet. I recommend that all my clients try Yoga, given the various benefits that this practice can bring to the body and mind. Yoga is perfect for any type of Intermittent Fasting diet, being a low-intensity training that can also be done with the most intensive diets.

Almost all people can perform the basic Yoga positions, and in addition to increasing the body's flexibility, they are perfect for regaining focus and starting the day well. Furthermore, since this activity is classified as low-intensity training, eating a meal before or after it is unnecessary. Instead, you can decide to wait a few hours before eating. This will allow to raise growth hormone levels and accelerate fat burning.

If you have never tried Yoga and are unsure if this is a suitable activity for you and are therefore reluctant to invest money for a course, I have decided to include some basic positions with this book.

Plus, there are tons of Youtube videos on the subject, so I'm sure you won't be short of learning material. Give it a try!

Cat Pose (Marjaryasana) / Cow Pose (Bitilasana)

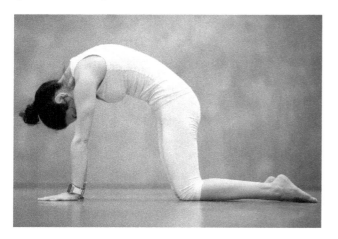

This is a gentle flow between two positions that mainly involves the back muscles and the spine. The starting position is on hands and knees with knees under the hips and hands under the shoulders, head in a neutral position. To move into Bitilasana, inhale and drop your belly towards the mat. Gaze up towards the sky, lifting chin and chest. Open your shoulders and relax, feeling the stretch on the spine. To transition into Marjaryasana, exhale and draw your belly to your spine while rounding the back towards the sky. Release your head towards the floor. Repeat the cycle up to 20 times.

Bridge Pose (Setu Bandha Sarvangasana)

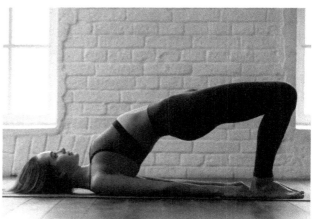

Lie on your back with knees bent and feet firmly on the floor. Place your arms on either side of your body with your palms facing down. Exhale as you lift your hips towards the sky while pressing both feet and arms into the floor. Roll your shoulders back. The only parts in contact with the floor must be your arms, feet, head, and upper back.

HAPPY BABY
(ANANDA BALASANA)

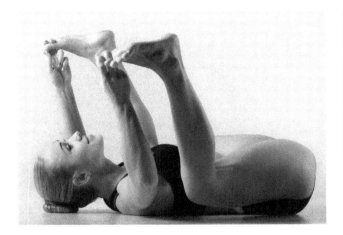

Lie on your back, and while exhaling, bend your knees into your belly. Inhale and grip your feet or toes with your hands. Open your knees slightly wider than your torso and bring them up toward your armpits. Be sure that each ankle is positioned over the knee.

CHILD'S POSE
(BALASANA)

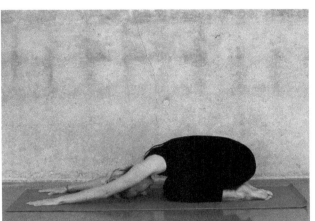

Come to your hands and knees on the mat. Slightly spread your knees and keep the top of your feet on the floor. Bend, bringing your forehead to the floor. It is essential to relax your spine, shoulders, and jaw. Stay as long as you like, feeling the nice stretch on your spine.

CORPSE POSE
(SAVASANA)

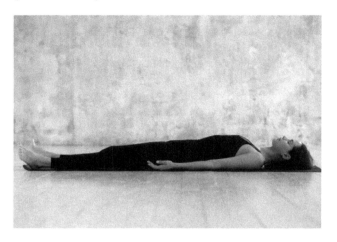

Lie on your back with legs and arms straight, palms facing upward. Stay as long as you like focusing on your breathing.

SUPINE SPINAL TWIST
(SUPTA MATSYENDRASAN)

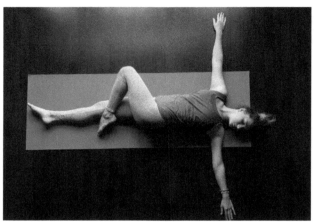

The Supine Spinal Twist stretches the back muscles and realigns and lengthens the spine giving more flexibility and endurance to the subject. Start lying down on your back and bring your arms in a T position, with the palms facing down. Next, bend your right knee over the left side of your body, twisting the spine and low back. Once in this position, use your left hand to push your right knee against the floor; you should feel your thigh and lower back stretching. Your gaze should look in the opposite direction of your knees or toward the ceiling. Keep your shoulders flat to the floor when twisting your body. Keep this position for 6-10 breaths before repeating it with the other side.

COBRA POSE
(BHUJANGASAMA)

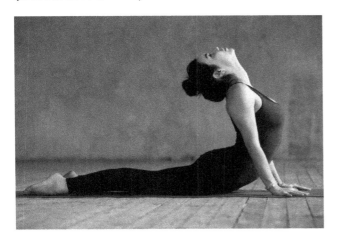

The cobra pose is ideal for beginners because of its simple execution. This pose increases mobility, especially for the back spine, and fortifies the spinal support muscles. In addition, since it opens the chest, it puts the body in a better position for full inhalation, which helps to release stress and pain.

To perform this position, start lying down on your stomach, legs extended, and the toes are pointing straight back and the top of your feet, thighs, and the pubis firmly into the floor. Spread your hands on the ground under the shoulders and push your torso up. On inhalation, lift your chest off the floor and straighten your arms. Next, lift the pubis toward the navel and narrow the hips points. When inhaling, your shoulders are moving back, opening your chest. Your shoulders should stay relaxed and the base of your neck soft, while your buttocks are firm but not harden. Keep this position from 10-30 seconds, breathing easily. After you fully exhale, relaxing your body and going down with your torso. Bend your elbows a little as your chest gets closer to the floor. Repeat this sequence from 5 to 10 times. At the end of this practice, you should feel much more light and relaxed!

THE DOWNWARD-FACING DOG
(ADHO MUKHA SVANASANA)

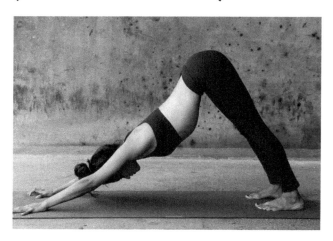

The downward-facing dog position works to strengthen the core and improve circulation. It is perfect for stretching, especially for the back, shoulders, hamstrings, and calves, and it helps tone your arm and leg.

Start this pose in an all-fours position, with the hands slightly forward your shoulders and spread your fingers. Firmly press your hands, applying the pressure on the edge of the palms and creating a suction cup in the middle (this status of your hands is called Hasta Bandha). Next, lift your hips to bring yourself into an upside-down V pose. In the beginning, keep your knees a bit bent when you adjust your back. Your Shoulders should blade down along the spine, and the base of your neck should stay relaxed. Maintaining your spine stretched, "walk your dog" by alternating bending and straightening your knees. With each exhalation, root down firmly through your hands; with each subsequent inhalation, send your hips back and up even more. Hold for anywhere from a few breaths to a few minutes, then release. For this position, remember to focus more to keep length in the spine than straight legs, so it's okay to keep your keens a bit bent if you need to feel more comfortable.

WARRIOR 1
(VIRABHADRASANA I)

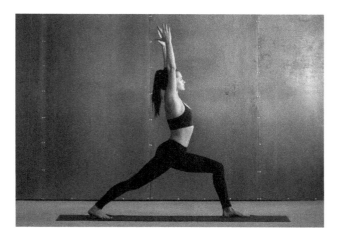

There are three variations for the Warrior Pose, and each of them can be performed to improve your tantric sex. I chose this one because it's ideal for stretching your muscles, and it also helps tone your thighs and butt. It will also improve your stamina and endurance that are always helpful for tantric love.

Start this position standing up straight. Then step your right foot back approximately 45° inward, while your front knee bend at 90° or slightly more. Next, straight your spins and drop your shoulders back while you raise your arms above your head. Your left leg should stay strong as you hold this position for 30 seconds or so. To release, unbend your front knee, centering the torso, and bring your arms down slowly. Repeat the pose bringing back your left leg this time.

PLOW POSE (HALASANA)

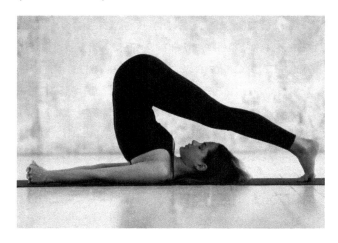

Halasana or Plow Pose is an inverted asana that stretches back and shoulders. This pose relaxes the nervous system and relieves stress and fatigue. Consider that this exercise is not a straightforward pose, and you may not get it right at the first attempt. The difficulty level is medium-hight, so it's better if you practice with the previous ones if you are a beginner, and for the first time, it's better if you check with someone that you are in the correct position.

To accomplish this pose, start lying flat on your back with the arms on your sides, hands with palms down, and then extend your legs. When inhaling, use your abdominal muscles to lift your hips and legs. Bring your torso perpendicular to the floor. Keeping your legs extended, slowly lower your toes until touching the floor. If you are struggling to touch the floor, don't worry, you just need some practice; put your toes as lower as you can, keeping the legs extended, and support your back with your hands. If you can reach the floor, then extend your arms and interlace your fingers, pressing your upper arms firmly into the floor. To have this position done correctly:

1. Your Torso is perfectly perpendicular to the floor

2. The legs are extended straight as much as you can

3. There is some space between your chin and the chest and softens your throat. Your eyes should gaze down toward your cheeks.

Once reached the position, hold the pose for up to five minutes.

To release, support your backs when returning your legs. Move slowly when rolling down, and if you need, you can bend your knees.

This pose is perfect for letting out your stress, and it's a good exercise for your stamina. It will help you to have better endurance and a relaxed mind.

SUPPLEMENTS

Supplements are a way to incorporate all the substances we need into our meals. The use of supplements is optional in Intermittent Fasting. Still, many of my clients have found benefits in using them to respect their macro goals, help the body adapt to this new lifestyle, and perform better during workouts. In this short section, I would like to provide you with a shortlist of supplements that may be useful to you during intermittent Fasting and their effects.

APPLE CIDER VINEGAR

Apple cider vinegar can be consumed during an intermittent fasting diet and has the characteristic of not breaking the fast. ACV contains a large amount of vitamins B1, B2, B6, and C, as well as biotin, folic acid, and pantothenic acid. The combination of these substances helps to support our body and improve the efficiency of the central nervous system. If you decide to consume ACV during your diet, I recommend drinking a high-quality, unrefined, pasteurized one to maintain unaltered nutritional values.

FISH OIL OMEGA-3S

Fish oil can indirectly help to lose weight as it can reduce appetite for some groups of people. Various studies have been conducted, and this effect, unfortunately, does not appear to be universal. For people classified as obese, the appetite reduction effect seems to be greater, while for people without weight problems, in some cases, the opposite effect has even been obtained.

Fish oil also seems to have the property of accelerating metabolism. Only one study has been carried out on this, but it has produced encouraging results. A group of healthy adults took 6g of fish oil per day for 12 weeks, seeing their metabolic rate increase by 3.8% on average.

PROTEIN POWDER

Unlike apple cider vinegar, protein shakes break the Fasting and should only be consumed during the eating window. Protein powder can be used to recover faster after workouts or to increase protein intake during meals. In addition, protein shakes can play a crucial role in weight loss. Unlike carbohydrates, proteins are digested more slowly and can increase the sense of satiety and reduce the production of ghrelin, the hormone that causes the feeling of hunger. The amount of pure protein that a person needs varies according to the physical activity performed, weight, and age. According to medical research, on average, 0.8g of protein is required for every kg of body weight.

This amount of protein can be achieved with a well-structured meal plan or by taking advantage of food supplements such as protein shakes.

CALCIUM AND VITAMIN D

When fasting, calcium and vitamin D are also helpful supplements to take. Calcium aids in regulating blood sugar, while vitamin D aids in the proper functioning of your entire body. Calcium may also help to prevent osteoporosis, a condition that causes bones to deteriorate. If your bones are weak or you are predisposed to osteoporosis, you can take this supplement on a daily basis.

B VITAMINS

B vitamins should be taken as a combination rather than as individual supplements when it comes to vitamins. B vitamins are responsible for the production of energy and fatty acids in your body. If this is the only supplement you take while fasting, you're missing out on one of the most important benefits of Fasting. This combination will help you gain energy while also improving your hormonal balance.

CREATINE

Creatine mimics and is made from the same substance found naturally in your body. Creatine is a substance that boosts energy and endurance, so consider including it in your supplement regimen. Creatine can help you feel great while fasting and also help you lose fat while building muscle mass.

~ CHAPTER 5 ~
# RECIPES

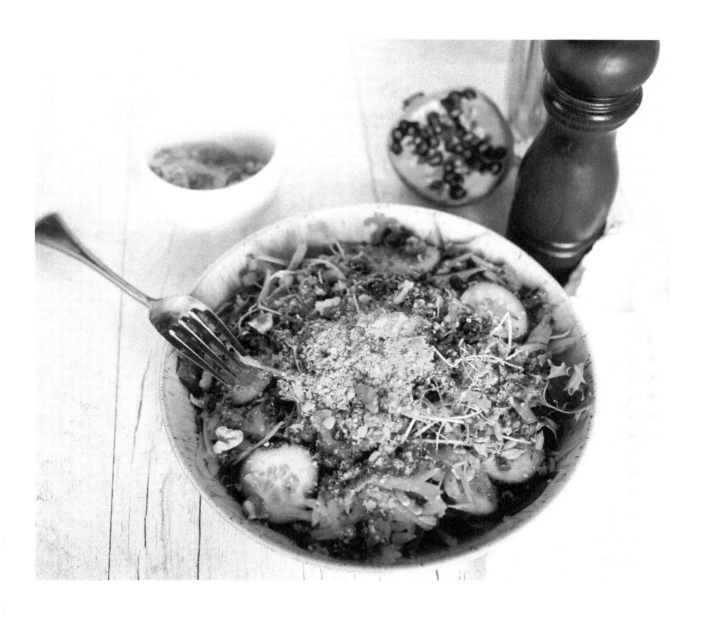

1. GRILLED PROSCIUTTO WRAPPED ASPARAGUS

INGREDIENTS:

- 8 asparagus spears
- 50g (1.7 oz) of prosciutto
- 1 tablespoon olive oil
- salt and black pepper to taste

TIME:
Prep. time: 5 min.
Cooking time: 10 min.
Servings: 2

NUTRITION (PER SERVING):
Calories: 56.2kcal
Protein: 4g
Cabs: 3g
Fat: 3.7g

DIRECTIONS:

1. Preheat the grill pan at medium temperature.
2. Cut off the tough woody ends of the asparagus and clean them with running water; then pat dry the spears with a paper towel.
3. Cut the prosciutto into eight slices and wrap each asparagus spear with a slice of prosciutto.
4. Brush each asparagus spear with some olive oil.
5. Season with salt and black pepper to taste.
6. When the grill pan is hot, place the asparagus on it, turning each spear frequently to cook all sides. The cooking time depends on the thickness of the asparagus; pierce with a fork to understand if they are ready; they should be tender but firm.

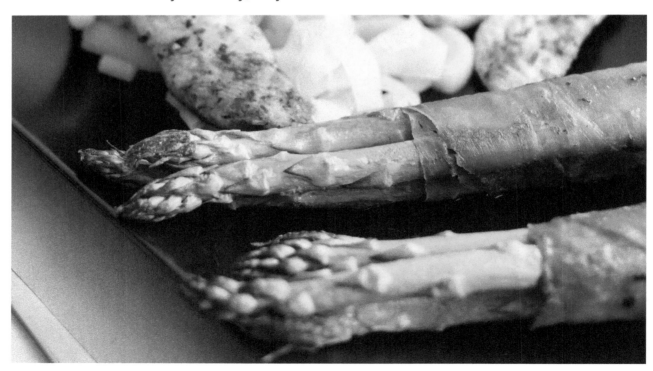

2. ZUCCHINI FRITTERS

INGREDIENTS:

✔ VEGETERIAN

- 1 medium zucchini, grated
- 1 large egg
- ¼ cup chopped fresh parsley
- ⅓ cup finely chopped yellow onion
- 1 tbsp mixed Italian herbs (basil, oregano, thyme, parsley)
- ⅓ cup grated Parmesan cheese
- ⅓ cup all-purpose flour
- ½ teaspoon baking powder
- Salt and black Pepper to taste
- 1 tbsp olive oil to fry with

TIME:
Prep. time: 10 min.
Cooking time: 10 min.
Servings: 2

NUTRITION (PER SERVING):
Calories: 204kcal
Protein: 12g
Cabs: 4.3g
Fat: 8g

DIRECTIONS:

1. Let the grated zucchini tossed with the salt sit for at least 10 minutes (the longer, the better). Then, squeeze the moisture out of zucchini using paper towels to remove all excess water. Removing most of the excess water is the key for crispy fritters!
2. Stir in the eggs, onions, garlic, and herbs. Then stir in the flour, Parmesan, and spices.
3. Heat the oil in a skillet over medium-high heat.
4. Once the oil is hot, drop about three tablespoons of batter per fritter in the skillet and cook for 4-5 minutes on each side until nicely browned.
5. Before serving, place the fritters on a paper towel to remove the excess cooking oil and pat the top with a sheet of kitchen paper.

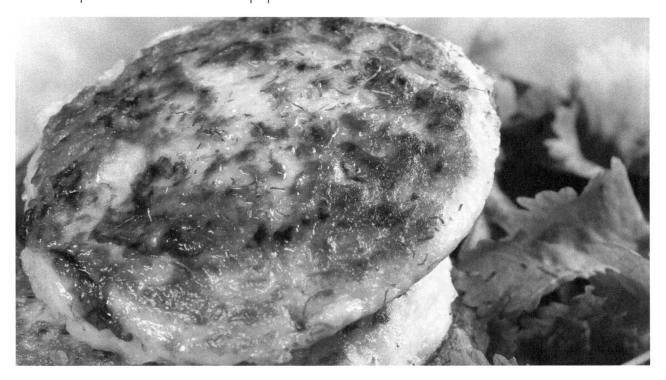

3. CAULIFLOWER AND GROUND BEEF HASH

INGREDIENTS:

- 6 oz. (150 g) bag frozen cauliflower, defrosted and drained
- 0.3 lb. (150 g) lean ground beef
- 1 cup of shredded cheddar cheese
- 1 tablespoon water or beef broth
- ⅓ cup finely chopped yellow onion
- ½ tsp of garlic powder
- 1 tbsp olive oil
- salt and black pepper to taste

TIME:
Prep. time: 5 min.
Cooking time: 20 min.
Servings: 2

NUTRITION (PER SERVING):
Calories: 304kcal
Protein: 31.9g
Cabs: 4.8g
Fat: 17.5g

DIRECTIONS:

1. Drain and chop the cauliflower into bite-size pieces.
2. Heat the oil in a skillet over medium heat.
3. When hot, cook the onions until they are translucent, then add the beef and cook it for about 5 minutes until browned.
4. Add in the pan the chopped cauliflower, garlic, water/broth, salt, and pepper. Cook and stir until the cauliflower is tender.
5. Add cheddar cheese on top of the cauliflower and beef mixture. Turn the heat to low and cover the pan with a lid, so the cheese fully melts before serving.

4. CHEESY TACO SKILLET

INGREDIENTS:

- 0.5 lb. (450 g) of minced beef
- 1 red pepper, chopped
- ⅓ cup sliced spring onions
- 2 cloves of garlic, crushed
- ¼ can (4 oz - 100 g) of black beans
- ½ can (7 oz - 200 g) of diced tomatoes
- 1 ½ cups of shredded cheddar cheese or Monterey Jack
- 1 tablespoon of taco seasoning
- 1 tablespoon extra virgin olive oil
- Chilli powder to taste
- Salt

TIME:
Prep. time: 5 min.
Cooking time: 20 min.
Servings: 2

NUTRITION (PER SERVING):
Calories: 342kcal
Protein: 21g
Cabs: 41g
Fat: 28g

DIRECTIONS:

1. Heat the oil in a large skillet over medium heat.
2. Add garlic and cook for about 2 minutes; add the chopped bell pepper and spring onions and cook it for about 5 minutes until tender. Remove the garlic.
3. Add the beef and cook it until browned, then add the taco seasoning and the chili—Cook for another couple of minutes.
4. Add diced tomatoes and black beans and cook it for about 10 minutes, stirring occasionally.
5. Place the shredded cheese on top of the mixture, turn the heat to low, and cover the pan with a lid. Let the cheese fully melt before serving.

5. LAMB SALAD WITH A THAI STYLE DRESSING

INGREDIENTS:

FOR SALAD:
- ½ lb. (230 g) lean lamb
- ½ cup bean sprouts
- ⅓ cup sliced spring onions
- 1 tablespoon vegetable oil
- 2 oz. (60 g) baby spinach
- 2 basil leaves
- 2 mint leaves
- 2 coriander leaves
- Salt

FOR DRESSING:
- ½ tablespoon soy sauce
- 1 tablespoon lime juice
- 1 teaspoon dark muscovado sugar
- 1 teaspoon fish sauce
- 1 tablespoon vegetable oil
- 1 red chili seeded and chopped

TIME:
Prep. time: 10 min.
Cooking time: 10 min.
Servings: 2

NUTRITION (PER SERVING):
Calories: 352kcal
Protein: 32g
Cabs: 0.4g
Fat: 18g

DIRECTIONS:

1. Wash and drain the beansprouts and the baby spinach.
2. Clean the basil, mint, and coriander leaves under running water, pat them with a paper towel until perfectly dry, and then cut them into small pieces.
3. Prepare the dressing by adding all the ingredients to a second bowl and whisk them with a fork.
4. Trim the lamb and cut it into thin strips.
5. Heat the oil in a frying pan or a wok and fry the lamb over high heat for about 3 minutes until browned.
6. Toss into the pan the sliced spring onion and stir fry for another 2 minutes.
7. Add the beansprouts and cook for 1 minute.
8. Move the ingredients from your pan into a bowl and add the baby spinach, the dressing, and the leaves cut into pieces.
9. Enjoy your salad until it's still warm!

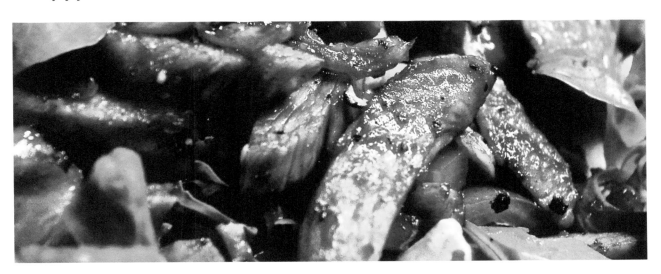

6. SAUSAGE & EGG CUPS

INGREDIENTS:

- 3 eggs
- ½ lb. (250 g) ground sausage
- ½ cup of shredded cheddar cheese or Monterey Jack
- ¼ teaspoon dried parsley
- ¼ teaspoon onion powder
- ¼ teaspoon garlic powder
- ¼ yellow onion diced
- ¼ cup baby spinach or rocket salad
- 1 strips bacon, cooked & crumbled
- ½ tomato diced
- Salt & Pepper to taste

TIME:
Prep. time: 15min.
Cooking time: 30min.
Servings: 2 (6 cups)

NUTRITION (PER SERVING):
Calories: 503kcal
Protein: 31g
Cabs: 3.1g
Fat: 37g

DIRECTIONS:

1. Preheat the oven to 350°F (180°C) and grease a 12 cup muffin pan.
2. In a bowl, mix sausage, salt, pepper, dried parsley, garlic powder, and onion powder until well combined.
3. Place the sausage mixture into the muffin pan, leaving some room in the middle for the eggs.
4. In a separate bowl, mix the eggs, salt, and pepper, then pour the egg mixture in the middle of each cup.
5. Top four cups with the bacon, four with the shredded cheddar cheese or Monterey Jack), four with the baby spinach or rocket salad, and four with the diced tomato.
6. Bake for 30 minutes and enjoy!

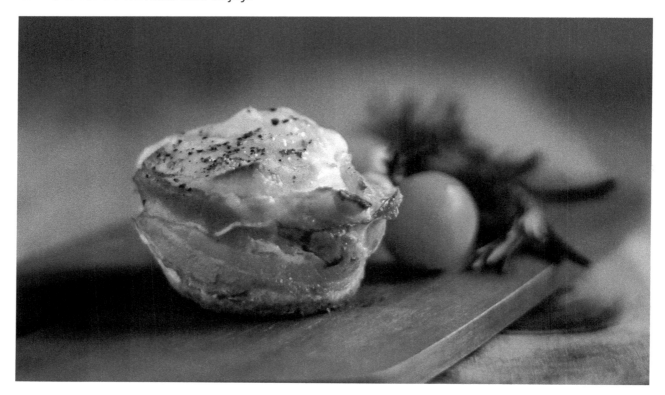

7. SMOKED SALMON & AVOCADO STACKS

INGREDIENTS:

- 2.6 oz. (75 g) smoked salmon, finely diced
- ½ ripe avocado, seed removed and diced
- 1 tbsp. chives, chopped
- Fresh or dried dill leaves

- 1 tbsps. fresh lemon juice
- 1 tablespoon olive oil
- Salt & Pepper to taste

TIME:
Prep. time: 15 min.
Cooking time: 0 min.
Servings: 2

NUTRITION (PER SERVING):
Calories: 106kcal
Protein: 5g
Cabs: 2.8g
Fat: 12g

DIRECTIONS:

1. In a bowl, mix salmon with chives, one teaspoon of lemon juice, and season to taste with salt and pepper.
2. Toss the avocado, olive oil, one teaspoon of lemon juice in a separate bowl, and season to taste with salt and pepper.
3. Place a ring mould in the center of the serving plate. Fill it with the avocado mixture and press down gently with the back of a spoon. Add a layer of the salmon mixture, pressing down gently to smooth the top.
4. Remove the mould and add some dill on the top for decoration. Serve chilled and enjoy!

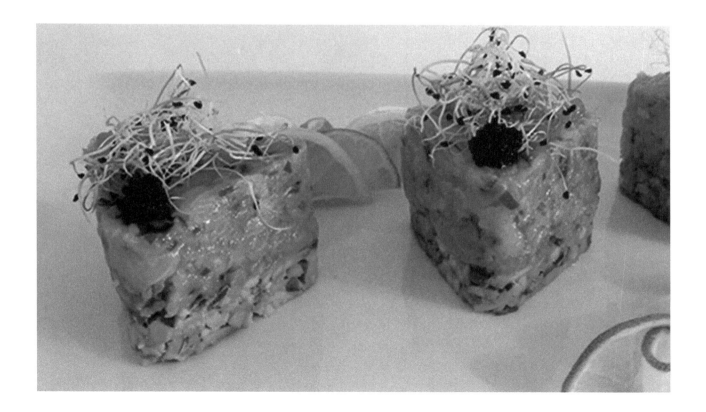

8. SESAME-SEARED SALMON

INGREDIENTS:

- 2 wild salmon fillets (about ½ lb - 230 g)
- 1 tbsps. sesame seeds
- 1 tbsps. toasted sesame oil
- ½ tbsps. cooking oil (I suggest avocado oil)
- Salt

TIME:
Prep. time: 5 min.
Cooking time: 10 min.
Servings: 2

NUTRITION (PER SERVING):
Calories: 277kcal
Protein: 25g
Cabs: 0g
Fat: 18g

DIRECTIONS:

1. Ensure the salmon fillets have no fishbones left, then wash the fish under running water and dry it with a paper towel.
2. Brush each salmon fillet with the sesame oil and season them with ½ teaspoon of sea salt.
3. Heat the oil in a large skillet over medium-high heat. Once the oil is hot, gently add the salmon fillets flesh side down. Cook for 3 minutes, then flip the salmon fillets and cook for another 3-4 minutes.
4. Remove the salmon from the pan and place it onto the plate. Brush each fillet with the reserved sesame oil and sprinkle with the sesame seeds—season to taste with salt and finally serve.

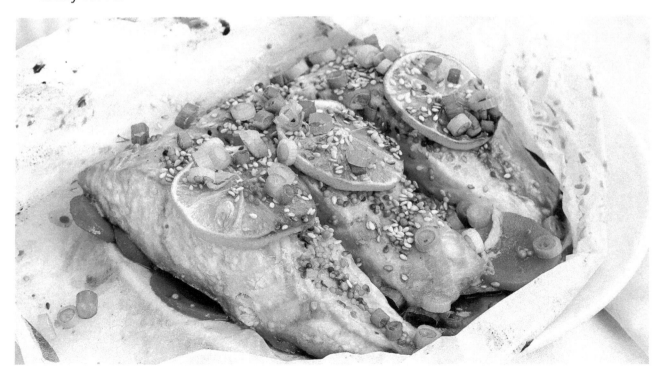

9. QUICK RATATOUILLE

INGREDIENTS:

✔ VEGETERIAN ✔ VEGAN

- ¼ large onion
- 1 clove of garlic
- 1 bell peppers
- ½ large eggplant
- 1 zucchini
- 3 large tomatoes
- 1 tsp salt

- 1 tsp olive oil
- 1 tsp black pepper
- 1 tsp dried or shredded fresh basil
- 1 tsp dried rosemary or 1 fresh sprig
- 1 large bay leaf

TIME:
Prep. time: 10 min.
Cooking time: 20 min.
Servings: 2

NUTRITION (PER SERVING):
Calories: 128kcal
Protein: 5g
Cabs: 15.5g
Fat: 3g

DIRECTIONS:

1. Cut all the vegetables into chunky pieces (about ½ inch cubes).
2. Heat the oil in a large pan over medium heat.
3. When the oil is hot, add the onions and the garlic and cook for a few minutes until translucent.
4. Add all the other ingredients and cook for about 15-20 minutes until the vegetables are tender and the tomatoes have mostly broken down. Stir frequently. You don't need to add water because the vegetables will release their liquids as they cook.
5. When the ratatouille is almost ready, you can adjust the flavor by adding one teaspoon of sugar if the flavor is a bit sour.
6. When ready, add salt and pepper to taste and remove the bay leaf before serving.

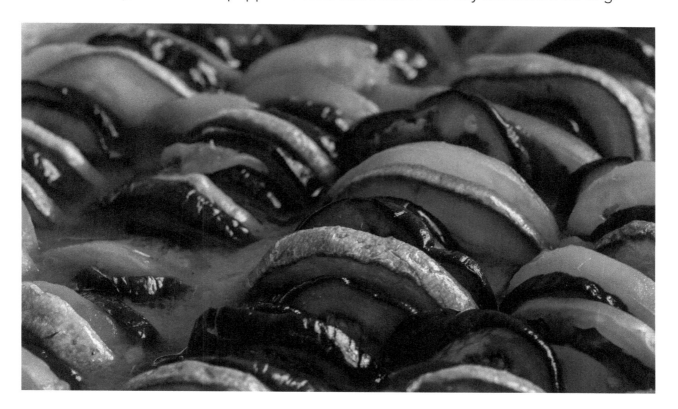

10. STUFFED PORTOBELLO MUSHROOMS

INGREDIENTS: ✔ VEGETERIAN

- 2 portobello mushrooms, the larger, the better
- 2 cups kale or spinach, chopped
- ¼ medium onion, chopped
- 2 cloves of garlic, minced
- ¼ cup breadcrumbs
- ¼ cup mozzarella cheese, shredded
- ¼ cup goat cheese, shredded
- 1 tbsp olive oil
- Salt and pepper to taste

TIME:
Prep. time: 10 min.
Cooking time: 10 min.
Servings: 2

NUTRITION (PER SERVING):
Calories: 220kcal
Protein: 15g
Cabs: 8.3g
Fat: 10g

DIRECTIONS:

1. Preheat the oven to 400°F (200°C).
2. Remove stems from mushrooms. Chop the stems and keep them on a side for the stuffing.
3. Place mushrooms onto a baking pan, cap-side down. Bake for 10 minutes until the water leaks out of them. Remove from the oven and, using paper towels, soak up excess water. Set aside.
4. Heat the olive in a skillet over medium heat. Add the chopped onion and garlic and saute for a few minutes until the onion is translucent. Add the kale or the spinach and cook for another couple of minutes until the leaves wilt.
5. Add goat cheese, mushroom stems, breadcrumbs, and season with salt and pepper to taste. Stir and cook for an additional couple of minutes.
6. Stuff the mushrooms with the mixture and top with mozzarella cheese.
7. Bake for 10 minutes until the cheese melts.

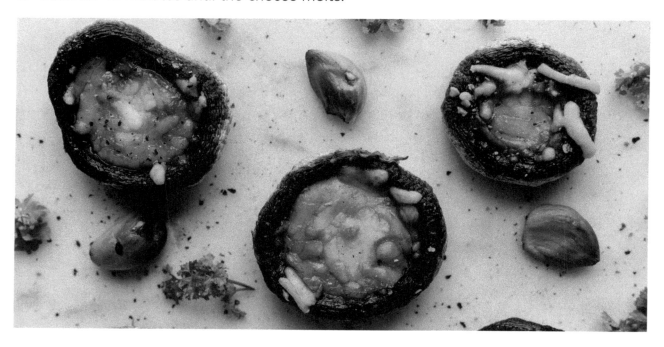

11. BOLOGNESE SOUP

INGREDIENTS:

- ¼ lb (125 g) pasta of your choice
- ¼ lb (125 g) steak mince
- ☐ lb (250 g) tomato passata
- 1 onion, finely chopped
- 1 large carrot, finely diced
- 1 celery stick, finely diced
- 1 clove of garlic, finely chopped
- ½ tbsp vegetable stock
- ½ tbsp smoked paprika
- 1 sprig of fresh thyme
- 1 oz (25g) Parmesan cheese, grated finely (plus extra for serving)
- 1 tsp olive oil
- ½ Litre water
- ¼ tsp black pepper
- 1 tsp salt

TIME:
Prep. time: 10 min.
Cooking time: 35 min.
Servings: 2

NUTRITION (PER SERVING):
Calories: 340kcal
Protein: 25g
Cabs: 14.2g
Fat: 10g

DIRECTIONS:

1. Heat the water in a stew pan over medium heat.
2. While the water warms up, heat the oil in a large non-stick pan over medium heat. When the oil is hot, add the onions and cook for a couple of minutes. Then, add the garlic, the carrots, and the celery and cook until the vegetables start to soften, stirring occasionally.
3. Add the meat and stir well to break it down as it cooks. Add tomato passata, paprika, thyme, pepper, and vegetable stock when the meat is browned. Add in the mixture the water that should now be boiling. My suggestion is to use a ladle and add the water carefully. Then add the salt. Cover the pan and simmer for 15 minutes.
4. Toss the pasta and cook for another 12-15 minutes. When the pasta is tender, add the Parmesan cheese, stir for 1-2 minutes, then ladle into bowls. Before serving, you can sprinkle over extra cheese if you like.
5. This dish is even better when cooked the previous day. You can store the soup in the fridge for up to seven days. Before putting the soup in the refrigerator, remove the thyme and chill the soup down to room temperature. Store it in the fridge covering the top with the lid or using some cling film. Reheat in the pan for a few minutes adding half a glass of water.

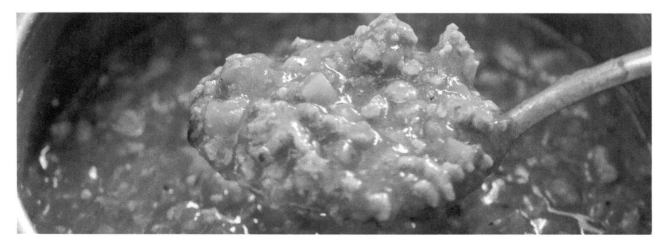

12. TURKEY-WALNUT SALAD

INGREDIENTS:

- ½ cups chopped cooked turkey
- ⅛ cup chopped toasted walnuts
- Mixed salad greens
- 1 celery ribs, sliced
- ¼ red onion, finely sliced
- ½ tsp lemon juice
- 1 tsp chopped fresh parsley
- ¼ tbsp Dijon mustard
- 1 tbsp dried cranberries
- ⅛ cup feta cheese, diced
- 1 tbsp olive oil
- ½ tsp ground pepper
- ½ tsp salt

TIME:
Prep. time: 10 min.
Cooking time: 0 min.
Servings: 2

NUTRITION (PER SERVING):
Calories: 286kcal
Protein: 24g
Cabs: 1g
Fat: 15g

DIRECTIONS:

1. Mix all the ingredients in a bowl and stir together. Serve it at room temperature.

13. CRISPY BLACK-EYED PEAS

INGREDIENTS: ✔ VEGETERIAN   ✔ VEGAN

- ½ can of black-eyed peas
- ¼ tsp ground coriander seed
- ¼ tsp chipotle chili powder
- ¼ tsp smoked paprika
- ¼ tsp garlic powder
- ¼ tsp salt
- ½ tbsp extra-virgin olive oil

TIME:
Prep. time: 10 min.
Cooking time: 50 min.
Servings: 2

NUTRITION (PER SERVING):
Calories: 99kcal
Protein: 7g
Cabs: 39g
Fat: 0g

DIRECTIONS:

1. Preheat the oven at 370° F (190° C).
2. Rinse the beans well with running water and spread them onto a paper towel to dry off.
3. Toss the beans into a bowl and mix well with all the seasonings.
4. Spray oil onto a baking pan and spread the beans mixed with the seasonings onto it.
5. Bake for about 50 minutes until they are deep brown and crispy. Stir the black-eyed peas every 10-15 minutes.

14. LEMONY GREEN BEANS

INGREDIENTS:

✔ VEGETERIAN   ✔ VEGAN

- ¼ lb (125 g) green beans washed and destemmed
- ½ lemon
- ½ tablespoon extra-virgin olive oil
- sea salt and black pepper to taste

TIME:
Prep. time: 2 min.
Cooking time: 15 min.
Servings: 2

NUTRITION (PER SERVING):
Calories: 48kcal
Protein: 1.5g
Cabs: 3.5g
Fat: 3g

DIRECTIONS:

1. Put a pan of salted water on to boil.
2. While the water is heating, trim the beans and wash them under running water.
3. Once the water in the pan is boiling, steam or boil the beans until tender.
4. Move the green beans to a large bowl and cover with olive oil.
5. Finely grate the lemon zest into the bowl, then cut the lemon in half and squeeze in the juice from one half onto the beans, making sure the lemon seeds don't get into the bowl.
6. Season with salt and pepper and mix everything.

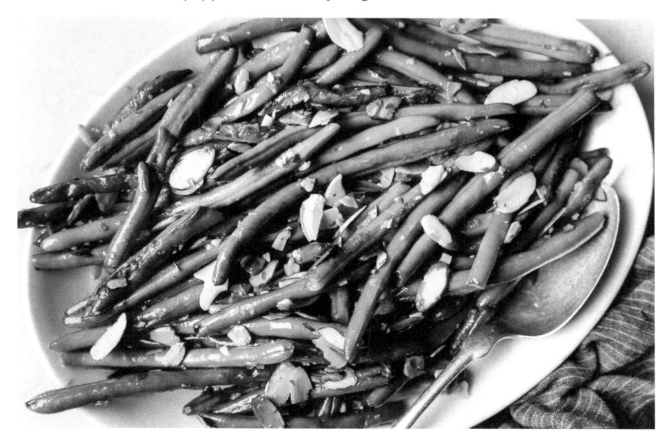

15. ROASTED ORANGE CAULIFLOWER

INGREDIENTS: ✔ VEGETERIAN ✔ VEGAN

- ½ large head of orange cauliflower
- ¼ lemon, juiced
- 1 tablespoon olive oil
- ½ tsp garlic powder
- ½ tsp onion powder
- Sea salt and black pepper to taste

TIME:
Prep. time: 10 min.
Cooking time: 25 min.
Servings: 2

NUTRITION (PER SERVING):
Calories: 40kcal
Protein: 3g
Cabs: 9g
Fat: 0.5g

DIRECTIONS:

1. Preheat the oven to 400°F (200°C).
2. Wash and cut cauliflower into florets—Pat dry with paper towels.
3. Place the florets in a baking pan and drizzle with olive oil and ½ lemon juice. Sprinkle it with garlic and onion powder and season with salt and pepper.
4. Cook in the oven for 20-25 minutes until golden brown. Stir cauliflower about halfway through roasting.

16. HONEY ROASTED BABY CARROTS

INGREDIENTS: ✔ VEGETERIAN

- 4 oz (120 g) baby carrots
- 1 tbsp olive oil
- ⅛ cup honey
- ¼ teaspoon ground cumin
- Salt and black pepper to taste

TIME:
Prep. time: 10 min.
Cooking time: 30 min.
Servings: 2

NUTRITION (PER SERVING):
Calories: 145kcal
Protein: 0.5g
Cabs: 18g
Fat: 7g

DIRECTIONS FOR THE PASTRY:

1. Preheat the oven to 425°F (220°F)
2. Place the carrots into a baking pan. Add olive oil, cumin, honey, and mix until evenly coated—season to taste with salt and black pepper.
3. Roast in the preheated oven for 30 minutes until just tender.

17. MEDITERRANEAN ROASTED

INGREDIENTS: ✔ VEGETERIAN   ✔ VEGAN

- 1 small zucchini
- 2 bell peppers
- 1 red onion
- 1 small eggplant
- 5 cherry tomatoes
- 1 tsp Italian herbs (basil, thyme, oregano, rosemary)

- 1 tbsp olive oil
- Salt and pepper to taste

TIME:
Prep. time: 10 min.
Cooking time: 20 min.
Servings: 2

NUTRITION (PER SERVING):
Calories: 120kcal
Protein: 2g
Cabs: 14g
Fat: 8g

DIRECTIONS:

1. Preheat the oven to 400°F (200°C)
2. Clean all the vegetables and dice them into similar chunks.
3. Add the chunks into a bowl. Add the oil, the herbs, and season to taste; then mix until each piece is well coated.
4. Transfer the chunks to a baking sheet and bake for 15-20 minutes until tender.
5. Serve them until warm.

18. BUTTERY BAKED CORN

INGREDIENTS: ✔ VEGETERIAN

- ¼ cup butter, room temperature
- ½ tbsp chopped parsley
- ¼ tbsp garlic powder
- 2 corn on the cob
- Salt to taste

TIME:
Prep. time: 5 min.
Cooking time: 35 min.
Servings: 2

NUTRITION (PER SERVING):
Calories: 286kcal
Protein: 4g
Cabs: 20g
Fat: 24g

DIRECTIONS FOR THE PASTRY:

1. Preheat the oven to 400°F (200°C).
2. Cut four pieces of kitchen foil large enough to contain a cob. Brush each cob with butter and sprinkle with parsley and garlic, then season to taste.
3. Place each cob on each piece of kitchen foil, seal the edges to form parcels, and bake for 35 minutes.

19. EGGPLANT PARMESAN PANINI

INGREDIENTS: ✔ VEGETERIAN

- 1 medium eggplant, sliced into ¼ -inch slices (~6 slices)
- 1 cup breadcrumbs
- 2 tbsp fresh oregano, chopped
- 1 tbsp fresh basil, chopped
- 1 tbsp fresh parsley, chopped
- 2 eggs
- 1 tbsp milk
- 2 cups fresh mozzarella cheese, thinly sliced

- 1 cup Parmesan cheese, grated
- 2 Italian ciabatta bread
- 2 cups marinara sauce
- 3 tablespoons pesto sauce jarred or homemade
- ¼ cup extra-virgin olive oil
- Sea salt
- ¼ tsp pepper

TIME:
Prep. time: 40 min.
Cooking time: 15 min.
Servings: 2

NUTRITION (PER SERVING):
Calories: 267kcal
Protein: 11.3g
Cabs: 41.3g
Fat: 8.5g

DIRECTIONS:

1. Sprinkle a lot of salt on each side of the eggplant slices. The salt will remove the excess water and improve the eggplant flavor. Place the slices between two sheets of paper towel and leave them for at least 30 minutes to dry off.
2. Meanwhile, in a bowl, combine breadcrumbs, Parmesan, pepper, and parsley.
3. In a shallow dish, whisk eggs and milk together.
4. Remove the excess salt from the eggplant slices using a clean paper towel. Make sure to remove as much salt as possible. Don't use water in this process because the eggplant must remain dry.
5. Dip the eggplant in egg, then in the crumbs mixture, pressing a bit against the crumbs to cover them well along all sides.
6. Heat 2 tbsp of extra-virgin olive oil in a nonstick skillet over medium heat. When the oil is hot, place half of your eggplant slices in the skillet and cook for 5 minutes, turning occasionally. The eggplant should become gold and crisp.
7. Transfer your cooked slices to paper towels to drain and repeat number 6 with the remaining oil and eggplant slices.
8. Warm the marinara sauce in a saucepan over low heat or in a microwave, add the fresh oregano and basil, then stir.
9. Meanwhile, heat a grill pan or a panini press to toast your bread. Cut your bread horizontally in the middle and place the two pieces face-down on the grill pan/panini press for 5 minutes.
10. Now it's time to assemble the panini. Spread some marinara sauce over one half of your bread, and spread onto the other half a teaspoon of pesto. Into your sandwiches, make 2-3 layers of eggplant, marinara sauce, mozzarella cheese, and pesto; then top your sandwich with the remaining slice of bread.
11. Grill sandwiches with the panini press for 5 minutes. Serve it warm!

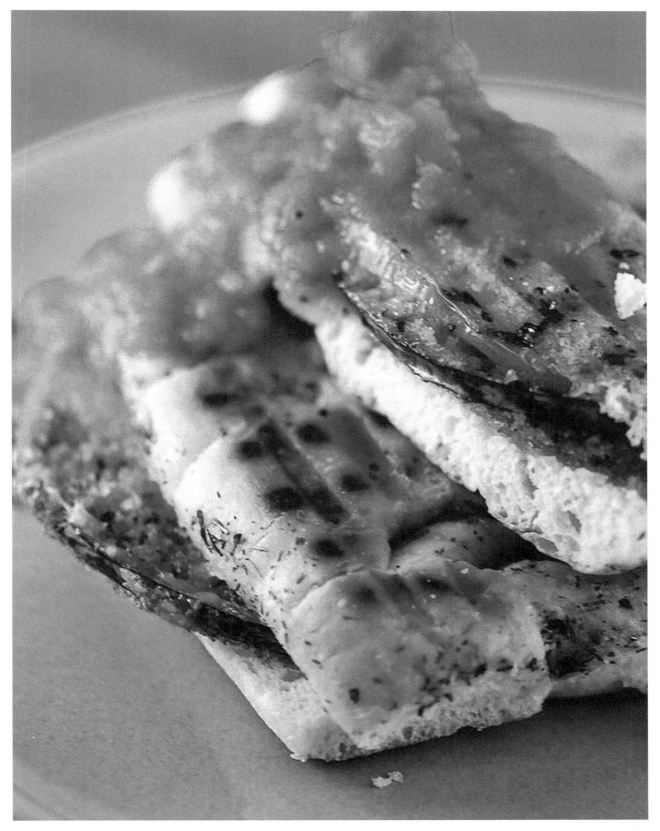

20. SPINACH AND CHEESE SAMOSAS

INGREDIENTS:

✔ VEGETERIAN

FOR SALAD:
- 1 cups flour
- ½ tsp salt
- ½ tsp vegetable oil plus extra for brushing
- water

FOR THE SEALING:
- ½ cup flour
- ¼ cup of water

FOR THE FILLING:
- ½ cup cream cheese
- ¼ cup feta cheese, diced
- ½ cup spinach, fresh or frozen
- ½ tsp garlic powder
- ¼ tsp black pepper
- ¼ tsp salt
- 1 medium egg

TIME:
Prep. time: 30 min.
Cooking time: 12 min.
Servings: 3 (9 samosas)

NUTRITION (PER SERVING):
Calories: 146kcal
Protein: 15g
Cabs: 12g
Fat: 10g

DIRECTIONS FOR THE PASTRY:

1. Preheat the oven at 400°F (200°C).
2. Add flour, salt, and vegetable oil in a bowl, then gently add water while mixing with your hands. Knead well until you get a soft dough. Cover it with a kitchen towel and let it sit for 30 mins. Cut the dough into three equal portions and form balls.
3. Take one ball and sprinkle some extra flour, then use a rolling pin to shape it into a circular shape. Repeat it for each ball, try to get shapes of similar size.
4. Pile the three circles spreading a lot of oil and flour between them. Roll the pile with the rolling pin until you get a 7" circle. Place the circle on a large baking pan and bake for a few minutes until the first layer puffs up.
5. Unbake the dough, cut the edges, making a square, and gently separate the sheets. The sheets should be soft, almost transparent, and shouldn't rip while separating.
6. Place each sheet on top of each other and cut into three equal strips. Now you have 9 strips for your samosas.

DIRECTIONS FOR THE SAMOSAS:

1. Preheat the oven at 400°F (200°C). Brush some oil on a baking sheet or baking pan.
2. First, we'll prepare the sealing for the samosa mixing the flour and the water until having a thick paste. Put it aside.
3. Cook the spinach, and when ready, place them between paper towels to dry them off. Make sure to squeeze out all the excess water from the spinach.
4. Combine cream cheese, feta cheese, spinach, garlic, pepper, and salt in a bowl.
5. Place a strip of samosa pastry vertically on a tray. Add two teaspoons of the mixture on the top-left corner and add one teaspoon of the flour and water paste on the bottom-right corner. Starting from the top-left corner, fold the samosa pastry over the filling, forming a triangle-shaped parcel. Once finished to shape, squeeze the samosa gently into your hands to improve the sealing. Continue this step for each strip you have.
6. Whisk the egg with some water and brush it on each samosa on both sides.
7. Place the samosas on a baking sheet and bake for up to 12 minutes until the samosas are golden and crispy. Serve immediately.

21. CRUNCHY CHILLI BABY CORN

INGREDIENTS: ✔ VEGETERIAN   ✔ VEGAN

FOR FRYING:
- ½ cup fresh baby corns
- 2 tbsp all-purpose flour or maida
- 2 tablespoons cornstarch (cornflour)
- 1 tbsp cornstarch (cornflour)
- ¼ teaspoon black pepper powder
- 1½ cups of water
- 1½ cups oil for frying (I suggest using corn oil or sunflower oil)

FOR SAUCE:
- ¼ cup chopped spring onion
- 2 cloves of garlic, finely chopped
- 1 tsp ginger, finely chopped
- ½ small green bell pepper, seeded finely chopped (optional)
- ½ tsp soy sauce
- ½ tbsp white vinegar or juice lemon
- 1 sliced red or green chili, to taste
- ¼ tsp sugar
- ½ tsp vegetable oil
- ½ tsp sesame Seeds

TIME:
Prep. time: 30 min.
Cooking time: 15 min.
Servings: 2

NUTRITION (PER SERVING):
Calories: 430kcal
Protein: 6g
Cabs: 17g
Fat: 33g

DIRECTIONS:

1. Boil the fresh baby corns for 5 minutes until tender
2. In a mixing bowl, add cornflour, all-purpose flour (or maida), black pepper powder, and mix well; then add some water to form a paste of medium-thick consistency. Add the boiled baby corn to the bowl and mix until well coated. Leave the corns into the bowl and heat the oil in a deep fry pan or a wok over medium heat.
3. When the oil is hot, fry the baby corn (to check if the oil is hot enough, drop a bit of pastry in the oil, if it starts to fry, the oil temperature is good enough). Cook the corns until they are golden brown and crispy.
4. Remove the corns and let them rest between two paper towels to remove the excessed oil. Meanwhile, heat 1 tsp of olive oil in a separated pan over medium heat, then add garlic, ginger, spring onion, chili, and green bell pepper. Cook over medium-high heat for 5 minutes, stirring frequently.
5. Lower the heat to medium and add the soy sauce and the white vinegar. Stir well. Lastly, add the crispy fried baby corn and stir for one minute more.
6. Plate the corn in a serving dish and sprinkle the sesame seeds on top before serving.

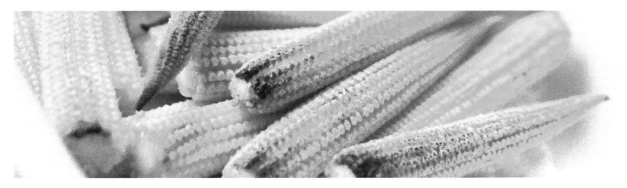

22. TASTY MARINATED TOFU

INGREDIENTS: ✔ VEGETERIAN

- 8 oz (225 g) extra-firm tofu
- 2 tbsp light soy sauce
- 2 tbsp rice vinegar
- ½ tbsp honey
- ½ tsp sesame oil
- 1 garlic cloves, minced
- ½ tbsp fresh grated ginger or ginger paste
- 1 tbsp vegetable oil

TIME:
Prep. time: 15 min.
(+ 1 hour or more to marinate)
Cooking time: 10 min.
Servings: 2

NUTRITION (PER SERVING):
Calories: 163kcal
Protein: 9g
Cabs: 7g
Fat: 10g

DIRECTIONS:

1. Cut the tofu into 1-inch cubes and place them on a flat surface, like a cutting board, with some paper towels in between. Cover the tofu with another layer of paper towels and set a baking sheet on top of it; then add something heavy, like a pan. Keep it pressing like this for 15 minutes.
2. While the tofu is pressing, you can prepare the marinade. In a bowl, combine soy sauce, rice vinegar, honey, garlic, and ginger.
3. Place the tofu in a large bowl and pour the marinade. Cover the bowl with some cling film and place it in the refrigerator. Let it marinate for at least 1 hour; my suggestion is to leave it overnight and cook it the next day for a better flavor!
4. To cook the tofu, heat 2 tbsp of vegetable oil in a large skillet over medium heat. If you prefer, you can skip the oil and use a non-stick grill pan instead. Cook the tofu cubes until browned on each side. Don't throw the marinade away!
5. Once the tofu is browned, pour the leftover marinade sauce into the pan and stir for a couple of minutes until the sauce is fully absorbed. Remove the tofu from heat and serve it with rice or vegetables. You can store any tofu leftover in a covered container for up to 3 days in the refrigerator. It's also good at room temperature with some salad and veggies.

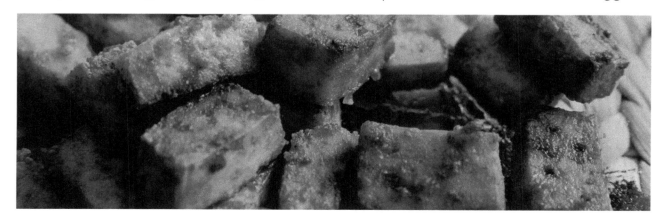

23. PARMESAN & FRESH HERBS ROASTED CAULIFLOWER BITES

INGREDIENTS:

✔ VEGETERIAN

- 1 large head cauliflower
- 2 small eggs
- ½ cup breadcrumbs
- ½ cup Parmesan cheese, grated
- 2 tsp Italian herbs (basil, thyme, oregano, rosemary)
- ¼ tsp garlic, powered
- 1 tbsp fresh lemon juice
- Salt and black pepper to taste
- Oil mister

TIME:
Prep. time: 10 min.
Cooking time: 35 min.
Servings: 2

NUTRITION (PER SERVING):
Calories: 362kcal
Protein: 23g
Cabs: 40g
Fat: 16g

DIRECTIONS:

1. Preheat the oven to 400°F (200°C).
2. Cut the cauliflower florets from the stem. Wash them under running water and place them onto a kitchen towel to let them dry.
3. In a large bowl, combine breadcrumbs, herbs, Parmesan cheese, and garlic powder.
4. Whisk the eggs in a small bowl adding salt and black pepper to taste.
5. Coat each floret first in the egg and then in the breadcrumbs mixture. Place them onto a baking pan with a baking sheet in between.
6. Spray some oil onto each floret and bake for 35 minutes until they get golden. Before serving, pour the lemon juice on top of the florets for a better flavor.

24. TURMERIC SOUR CREAM TILAPIA WITH PARMESAN CRUST

INGREDIENTS:

✔ VEGETERIAN

- ½ lb (225 g) tilapia fillets
- 3 oz (85 g)sour cream
- ⅛ cup parmesan cheese, grated
- ½ tbsp fresh parsley, chopped
- ⅛ cup breadcrumbs
- ⅛ tbsp garlic powder
- ½ tbsp butter or margarine softened
- ½ tsp turmeric powder
- Salt and pepper to taste

TIME:
Prep. time: 5 min.
Cooking time: 35 min.
Servings: 2

NUTRITION (PER SERVING):
Calories: 264kcal
Protein: 27g
Cabs: 13g
Fat: 20g

DIRECTIONS:

1. Preheat the oven at 350°F (180°C) and spray a large baking pan with oil.
2. Season the fillets with salt and pepper and put them in a foil-lined shallow baking pan in one single layer.
3. Add butter or margarine softened in a bowl, then add sour cream, garlic powder, turmeric powder, parsley, and season with salt and pepper. Stir together and add the parmesan cheese. Stir well and pour the cream all over the fillets. Sprinkle the top breadcrumbs.
4. Bake for 30 minutes until the surface becomes nicely golden and the fish flakes.

25. TILAPIA WITH SAVORY HERB BUTTER

INGREDIENTS:

- ½ lb (225 g) tilapia fillets
- ⅛ cup butter or margarine softened
- ¼ tsp garlic powder
- ½ tbsp mixed Italian herbs (basil, oregano, thyme, parsley)
- ¼ tsp ground mustard
- ¼ fresh lemon
- Salt and Pepper to taste
- Oil for the baking pan

TIME:
Prep. time: 5 min.
Cooking time: 12 min.
Servings: 2

NUTRITION (PER SERVING):
Calories: 227kcal
Protein: 27g
Cabs: 13g
Fat: 20g

DIRECTIONS:

1. Preheat the oven at 350°F (180°C) and spray a large baking pan with oil.
2. Season the tilapia fillets with salt and pepper and put them on the baking pan.
3. In a bowl, mix butter, garlic powder, Italian herbs, and ground mustard until well combined, then pour the mixture over the fish and spread with the back of a spoon.
4. Bake for 12 minutes until the fish flakes easily with a fork.
5. Put the fish on dishes, squeeze the half lemon juice on top of each fillet and serve.

26. LEMON SHRIMP IN PARMESAN CREAM

INGREDIENTS:

- ¼ lb (120 g) jumbo-sized shrimp
- ½ tbsp butter
- ½ tbsp fresh ginger, minced
- 1 clove of garlic, minced
- 1 cup half and half (or milk)
- ¼ cup fresh Parmesan cheese, grated
- ⅛ cup chopped fresh parsley
- Juice of ½ fresh lemon
- ¼ lemon for garnish, finely sliced

TIME:
Prep. time: 10 min.
Cooking time: 10 min.
Servings: 2

NUTRITION (PER SERVING):
Calories: 205kcal
Protein: 25g
Cabs: 9g
Fat: 8g

DIRECTIONS FOR THE PASTRY:

1. Heat the butter in a large skillet over medium-high heat until the butter has melted. Add the shrimp and cook for 1-2 minutes until pink. Remove the shrimp from the pan and set it aside.
2. In the same pan, add garlic and ginger to the remaining butter and fry for 1 minute. Turn the heat to low-medium heat and add half and half (or milk). Season with salt and pepper to taste and bring the sauce to a boil, then add the parmesan cheese and let it melt, allowing the sauce to simmer for about 2 minutes until thicker.
3. Add the shrimp back into the pan and pour in the lemon juice. Sprinkle the parsley and add on top the lemon slices. Pop the lid on the pan and let it cook for 1 minute more.
4. Serve over pasta, rice, or steamed vegetables.

27. COCONUT CURRIED COD

INGREDIENTS:

- ½ lb cod fillet, cut into bite-sized chunks
- 1 tsp garam masala curry
- 1 tsp turmeric
- 1 tsp paprika
- 2 tbsp olive oil
- 1 yellow onion, finely sliced
- 2 garlic cloves, finely sliced
- 1-inch ginger, grated
- 1 red chili seeded and chopped
- 1 cup vegetable broth
- 1 can - 13.5 fl oz (400ml) coconut milk
- ½ cup fresh cilantro leaves, chopped
- ½ fresh lemon
- Kosher salt and fresh cracked pepper to taste
- 1 cup basmati rice, boiled (for serving)
- 2 naan bread (optional)

TIME:
Prep. time: 10 min.
Cooking time: 20 min.
Servings: 2

NUTRITION (PER SERVING):
Calories: 655kcal
Protein: 27g
Cabs: 25g
Fat: 50g

DIRECTIONS:

1. In a bowl, combine curry, turmeric, and paprika. Use half of the spice mixture to coat the fish and season with salt and pepper. Set the fish aside.
2. Heat the oil in a lidded frying pan over medium heat. Add the onion, garlic, ginger, chili and cook for a few minutes until the onion gets translucent. Add vegetable broth and the remaining spice mixture and let it cook for 1 minute to allow the species to release their flavor.
3. Pour in the coconut milk, bring to a boil, cook for 5 minutes to reduce slightly, and add the cod. Cover the pan with the lid and let it cook for about 5 minutes until the fish flakes with a fork. Add the cilantro leaves and season with salt and pepper to taste. Serve with basmati rice and naan bread.

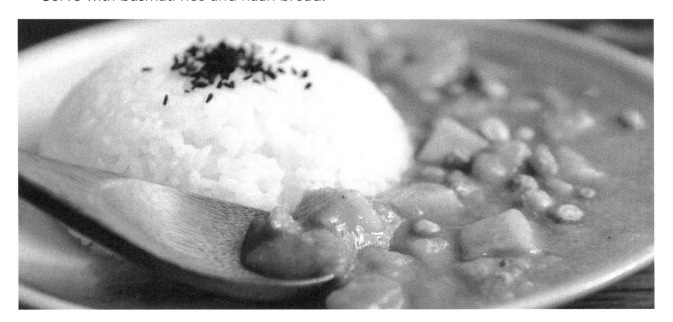

28. CAJUN SEASONED SALMON

INGREDIENTS:

- 2 wild salmon fillets (about ¾ lb - 350 g)
- 2 tbsp taco seasoning, possibly sodium-free
- ¼ cup water
- ½ lb (225 g) head cauliflower, finely chopped
- ½ lb (225 g) head broccoli (about 1 lb), finely chopped
- 5 medium fresh tomatoes, diced
- ¼ tsp garlic powder
- 2 tbsp olive oil
- Salt to taste

TIME:
Prep. time: 10 min.
Cooking time: 30 min.
Servings: 2

NUTRITION (PER SERVING):
Calories: 410kcal
Protein: 42g
Cabs: 11g
Fat: 25g

DIRECTIONS:

1. Preheat the oven to 350°F (180°C). Mix taco seasoning with ½ cup of water in a bowl and use the mixture to coat the salmon fillets all over. Place the salmon fillets in a baking pan and bake for 13 minutes.
2. While the salmon is cooking, let's prepare the vegetables. Cauliflower, broccoli, and onion should be finely chopped; each piece should be rice-size. I suggest chopping them using a food processor.
3. Heat 2 tbsp of oil in a large skillet over medium heat. When the oil starts shimmering, add broccoli and cauliflower and sprinkle with the garlic powder. Cook for 5 minutes, occasionally stirring, until they get tender.
4. Once the vegetables are cooked, put them into a bowl. Add diced fresh tomatoes, parsley, 1 tbsp of oil, and season with a pinch of salt. Mix well and place the mixture into a plate.
5. Remove the salmon from the oven and place it on the plate on top of vegetables and serve!

29. TUNA & WHITE BEAN SALAD

INGREDIENTS:

- 1½ tbsp lemon juice
- 1 tbsp extra-virgin olive oil
- ⅛ tsp salt
- Pepper to taste
- ½ garlic clove, minced
- ⅛ cup chopped red onion
- 3 oz (100 g) light tuna can in water, drained and flaked
- 10 oz (260 g) white cannellini beans can rinsed

TIME:
Prep. time: 10 min.
Cooking time: 0 min.
Servings: 2

NUTRITION (PER SERVING):
Calories: 140kcal
Protein: 16.9g
Cabs: 7.5g
Fat: 23g

DIRECTIONS:

1. Put all the ingredients in a bowl and mix well.
2. Serve!

30. CREAMY GARLIC KING PRAWNS WITH GOAT CHEESE

INGREDIENTS:

- 8.5 oz (250g) king prawns, peeled and cleaned
- 1 tbsp butter
- 2 cloves of garlic, minced
- ½ tsp paprika powder
- ⅛ cup goat cheese. crumbled
- 1 tbsp fresh parsley, chopped
- ¼ fresh lemon
- Salt and pepper to taste

TIME:
Prep. time: 10 min.
Cooking time: 5 min.
Servings: 1

NUTRITION (PER SERVING):
Calories: 470kcal
Protein: 60g
Cabs: 27g
Fat: 7g

DIRECTIONS:

1. In a large skillet, melt the butter over medium heat. Add the garlic and after a couple of minutes, add the king prawns too. Let it cook for one minute before adding the paprika powder. Cook for another minute; then turn the prawns and cook the other side for another 2 minutes.
2. When the prawns are cooked through, turn off the heat and add the crumbled goat cheese and the parsley to the pan. Stir to combine altogether and plate. Squeeze the juice of a slice of lemon on top before serving.

31. PORK CHOPS WITH BLOODY MARY TOMATO SALAD

INGREDIENTS:

- 1 tbsp olive oil
- ½ head green-leaf lettuce leaves torn
- 1 tsp Worcestershire sauce
- ¼ tsp tabasco
- 1 tbsp red wine vinegar
- ¼ tsp celery seeds
- Salt and pepper
- ½ pint (140 g) cherry tomatoes, halved
- 2 celery stalks, thinly sliced
- ¼ small red onion, sliced
- 2 bone-in pork chops

TIME:
Prep. time: 10 min.
Cooking time: 15 min.
Servings: 2

NUTRITION (PER SERVING):
Calories: 400kcal
Protein: 39g
Cabs: 8g
Fat: 23g

DIRECTIONS:

1. Heat grill pan to medium-high. Season pork chops with salt and pepper.
2. Mix oil, vinegar, tabasco, Worcestershire sauce, salt, tomatoes, celery seeds, onion, and parsley in a bowl.
3. Grill the pork chops for about 6 minutes per side until golden brown.
4. Serve pork chops and tomato salad.

32. HONEY SESAME SALMON IN FOIL

INGREDIENTS:

- 2 salmon fillets
- ½ tbsp lemon juice
- ⅓ cup spring onion, sliced
- ¼ tbsp sesame seeds
- 1 tbsp light soy sauce
- ¼ tbsp rice wine vinegar
- ¼ tbsp butter
- ¼ tbsp garlic, powder
- ¼ tbsp paprika, powder

- ¼ tbsp ginger, minced
- ½ tbsp sesame oil
- ½ tbsp fresh lemon juice
- ½ tbsp butter, melted
- 1 tbsp honey
- Salt and black pepper to taste

TIME:
Prep. time: 15 min.
Cooking time: 12 min.
Servings: 2

NUTRITION (PER SERVING):
Calories: 250kcal
Protein: 22g
Cabs: 12g
Fat: 13g

DIRECTIONS:

1. Preheat the oven to 350°F (180°C).
2. Prepare four sheets of kitchen foil big enough to fold over the salmon and seal to create a packet. Place them on a baking tray.
3. Place a small sauce over medium heat; add the soy sauce and the butter and whisk until well combined. Take off the heat, and add lemon juice, garlic, vinegar, paprika, sesame oil, ginger, and sesame seeds.
4. Season each fillet of salmon to taste with salt and pepper and place them on each sheet of kitchen foil. Shape the kitchen foil pulling up the edges and folding the sides; it must contain the liquid without leaking. Gently pour the honey-sesame mixture over each salmon, then seal the kitchen foil to close the package.
5. Bake the salmon and cook for 12-14 minutes, depending on the thickness size of your fillets.
6. Remove the salmon from the oven and carefully open the kitchen foil. Grill the salmon over medium heat or place it under the broiler for 3-5 minutes to caramelize the top. Keep your eye on it so it doesn't burn, and be careful not to overcook the salmon.
7. Garnish with the sliced spring onion and serve until warm!

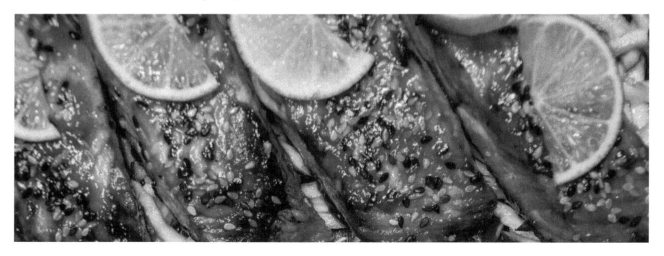

33. TUSCAN BUTTER SALMON

INGREDIENTS:

- 2 salmon fillets
- 2 cups baby spinach leaves
- 4 oz (125 g) cherry tomatoes, cleaned and cut in halves
- 1 cloves garlic, finely diced
- ¼ yellow onion, finely diced
- 1 tbsp butter
- 1 cup half and half or single cream
- ¼ cup fresh grated Parmesan cheese
- 1 tsp chopped fresh parsley plus more for garnish
- 1 tsp chopped fresh basil plus more for garnish
- ¼ fresh lemon
- 1 tbsp extra-virgin olive oil
- Salt and black pepper to taste

TIME:
Prep. time: 5 min.
Cooking time: 20 min.
Servings: 2

NUTRITION (PER SERVING):
Calories: 582kcal
Protein: 50g
Cabs: 30g
Fat: 35g

DIRECTIONS:

1. Heat the oil in a large skillet over medium-high heat. Season the salmon all over with salt and black pepper and sear in the pan, flesh-side down. Cook for 4-5 minutes on each side, then flip over and cook for another 4 minutes. When golden, remove the salmon from the pan and set it aside.
2. Reduce the heat to low and add butter. Once the garlic is melted, add garlic, onion and stir for about 1-2 minutes until the onion is translucent. Add the cherry tomatoes and cook for about 5 minutes until the tomatoes begin to soften.
3. Add the spinach and cook until spinach begins to wilt, then add half and half (or single cream), Parmesan cheese, herbs, and bring the mixture to a simmer. Let it cook for 3 more minutes while stirring occasionally.
4. Replace the salmon in the skillet, spoon over the sauce, and let it cook for 2 minutes.
5. Place the salmon onto plates and pull some sauce over it. Garnish with extra herbs and squeeze the lemon on top of each fillet before serving.

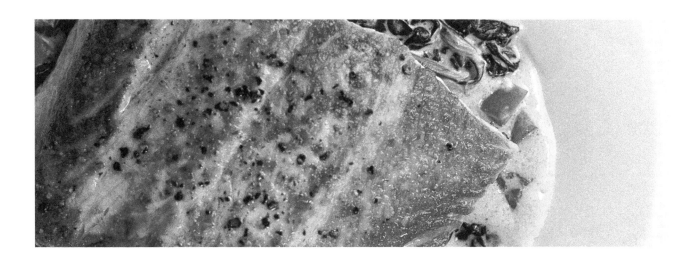

34. MAHI-MAHI COCONUT CURRY STEW

INGREDIENTS:

- 2 skinless mahi-mahi fillets
- ¼ cup fresh lemon juice
- ¼ cup vegetable oil
- 2 garlic cloves, peeled
- ¼ shallots, diced
- 1 cups large carrots, peeled and Shredded
- ¼ cup sliced spring onions
- 1 red chili pepper, sliced

- ½ tbsp fresh curry leaves
- ½ tbsp kaffir lime leaves
- ½ tbsp fresh ginger, minced
- 1 cups fennel bulb-halved, cored, and sliced
- ¼ tbsp curry powder
- 1 can - 7 fl oz (200ml) coconut milk
- Salt to taste

TIME:
Prep. time: 10 min.
Cooking time: 35 min.
Servings: 2

NUTRITION (PER SERVING):
Calories: 294kcal
Protein: 29g
Cabs: 23g
Fat: 15g

DIRECTIONS:

1. Place the mahi-mahi fillets in a large dish. Pour the lemon juice over the fillets and season with salt. Cover with cling film and refrigerate for at least 30 minutes.
2. Heat the oil in a large casserole over medium heat. When the oil is shimmering (but not smoking), add the garlic cloves and cook for about 2 minutes. Add shallots and spring onions and cook for about 2 minutes until the shallots get translucent, stirring occasionally. Add red chili pepper, ginger, curry leaves, lime leaves and cook for 2 minutes.
3. Add the fennel, carrots, and curry powder and season with salt. Let it cook for about 5 minutes, stirring occasionally. Add the coconut milk and bring to a simmer. Reduce the heat to low and let it cook for 10 minutes longer until the carrots are tender.
4. Add the mahi-mahi fish into the casserole and any juices accumulated in the dish. Cover the casserole with the lid and keep it cooking for about 15 minutes, shifting the fish occasionally.
5. Once the fish is cooked, transfer the stew into bowls for serving using a ladle and serve.

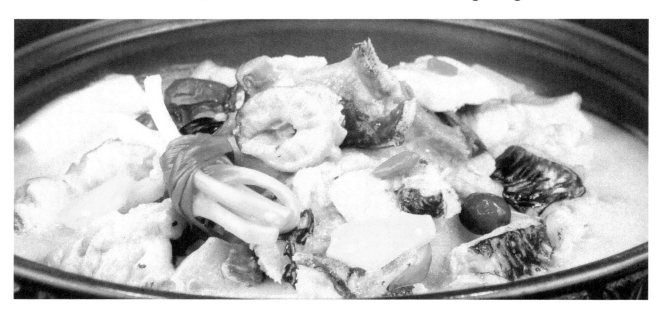

35. ROASTED PORK TENDERLOIN WITH BRUSSELS SPROUTS AND BUTTERNUT SQUASH

INGREDIENTS:

- 1 lb (450 g) pork tenderloin, trimmed
- 1 sprig of fresh thyme
- 1 garlic cloves, peeled
- 2 cups Brussels sprouts, trimmed and halved
- 2 cups butternut squash, diced
- 1 tbsp rapeseed oil
- ¼ fresh lemon juice
- Salt and pepper to taste

TIME:
Prep. time: 5 min.
Cooking time: 35 min.
Servings: 2

NUTRITION (PER SERVING):
Calories: 405kcal
Protein: 48g
Cabs: 25g
Fat: 17g

DIRECTIONS:

1. Preheat the oven to 400°F (200°C).
2. Season the tenderloin all over with salt and pepper. Heat 1 tbsp of oil in a large cast-iron skillet. When the oil shimmers, add the tenderloin into the pan and cook until golden, up to 10 minutes total. Then transfer to a plate and set them aside.
3. Add the remaining 1 tbsp rapeseed oil in the skillet, wait until it shimmers, then add the cloves of garlic and the thyme. Let it cook for one minute, then add the Brussels sprouts and the butternut squash. Season with a pinch of salt and pepper. Cook for 5 minutes, until browned, stirring occasionally.
4. Place pork and vegetables onto a baking pan with a kitchen foil sheet in between and transfer into the oven. Roast for 15-20 minutes, depending on the thickness of the tenderloin.
5. Remove from the oven and allow the pork to rest for 5 minutes. Place the pork tenderloin and the vegetables on a plate. Squeeze half lemon juice on top and serve!

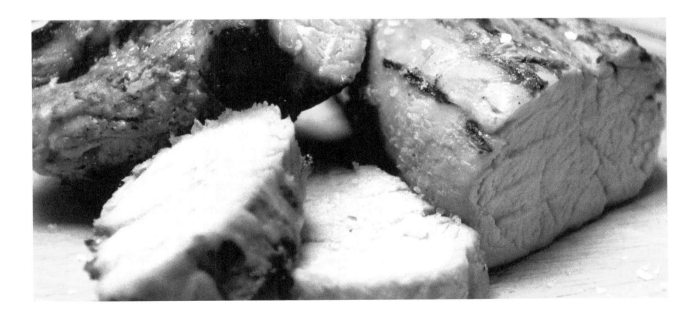

36. LENTIL, SPINACH AND TOMATO SALAD

INGREDIENTS: ✔ VEGETERIAN ✔ VEGAN

- 4 oz (125 g) dried green lentil, rinsed
- ¼ lime juice
- ¼ lemon juice
- ½ tbsp cider vinegar (or white wine)
- 1 tbsp extra-virgin olive oil

- ½ tsp ground cumin
- 4 oz (125 g) cherry vine tomato, halved
- 1 oz (30 g) baby spinach, washed and dried
- ½ small garlic clove, crushed
- ½ tiny red onion, sliced

TIME:
Prep. time: 5 min.
Cooking time: 20 min.
Servings: 2-3

NUTRITION (PER SERVING):
Calories: 150kcal
Protein: 11g
Cabs: 25g
Fat: 5g

DIRECTIONS:

1. Boil the lentils following the directions on the pack. Drain, rinse well, then drain one last time.
2. Mix all the ingredients and serve!

37. CHICKEN WITH FRIED CAULIFLOWER RICE

INGREDIENTS:

- 6 cups of diced cauliflower
- 3 tbsp sesame oil
- 0.6 lb (280 g) chicken breast, chopped into small cubes
- 3 medium carrots, diced
- ½ onion, diced
- 2 garlic cloves

- 2 tbsp fresh ginger, minced
- 1½ cup frozen sweet peas
- 2½ tbsp low sodium soy sauce
- 1 tbsp tamari sauce
- 1½ tsp sriracha sauce
- Sesame seeds for garnish

TIME:
Prep. time: 10 min.
Cooking time: 30 min.
Servings: 2

NUTRITION (PER SERVING):
Calories: 160kcal
Protein: 23g
Cabs: 16g
Fat: 6g

DIRECTIONS:

1. Put cauliflower in a blender. Blend until the pieces are the same size as a grain of rice. Set aside.
2. Heat a wok over medium heat.
3. In the wok, add a tablespoon of sesame oil and the chicken.
4. Cook the chicken for 4-5 minutes, making sure it is well browned on all sides. Remove the chicken from the wok and set it aside.
5. Add another tablespoon of oil to the wok and the chopped onions. Cook for about 2 minutes.
6. Add garlic ginger, and carrots and cook for another 4 to 5 minutes.
7. Finally, add the cauliflower rice, peas, soy sauce, tamari sauce, and sriracha sauce—Cook for about 2 minutes.
8. Add the chicken again and mix—Cook over medium heat for another minute.
9. Garnish with sesame seeds and serve hot.

38. TURKEY TACOS

INGREDIENTS:

- ½ small red onion, sliced
- ½ lb. extra-lean ground turkey
- ½ tbsp sodium-free taco seasoning
- 1 tsp oil
- ½ cup water or broth
- 4 whole-grain corn tortillas
- ⅛ cup sour cream

- ¼ cup Mexican cheese, shredded
- ½ avocado, sliced
- ½ cup lettuce, chopped
- 1 medium fresh tomatoes, sliced

TIME:
Prep. time: 0 min.
Cooking time: 25 min.
Servings: 2

NUTRITION (PER SERVING):
Calories: 474kcal
Protein: 25g
Cabs: 30g
Fat: 32g

DIRECTIONS:

1. Heat the oil in a large pan over medium heat. Add the onion and cook for 5 minutes until translucent. Then add the turkey and cook for 5 more minutes until browned while breaking it up with the spoon. Add the taco seasoning and 1 cup of water (or broth). Let it simmer for up to 10 minutes, letting the liquid reduce almost entirely.
2. Take a large non-stick pancake pan or a large casserole pan to warm the tortillas. Heat the pan over medium heat; when it's hot, toss one tortilla (or more if they fit) and warm it on each side for about 30 seconds - 1 minute.
3. Place 1-2 leaves of lettuce in each tortilla and 2 slices of tomato. Then fill with turkey and onion, and top with sour cream, avocado, and cheese.

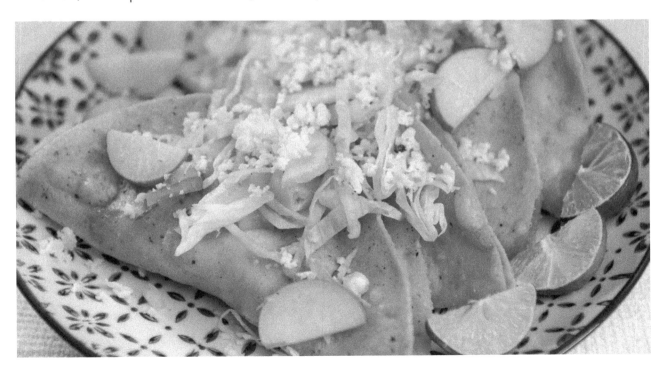

39. ASIAN-STYLE CHICKEN SALAD

INGREDIENTS:

- 0.5L (2 cups) water
- ½ brown onion
- 1 chicken breast
- 1 small carrot peeled, cut into sticks
- 2.5 oz (75 g) snow peas, trimmed and sliced
- ½ red bell pepper, deseeded and sliced

- ¼ Chinese cabbage (wombok), hard core removed, finely shredded
- 1 green shallot, thinly sliced
- ¼ cup fresh coriander leaves
- 1 tbsp lime juice
- ½ tbsp fish sauce
- 1 tsp brown sugar
- ½ red chili, chopped

TIME:
Prep. time: 15 min.
Cooking time: 10 min.
Servings: 2

NUTRITION (PER SERVING):
Calories: 200kcal
Protein: 34g
Cabs: 14g
Fat: 3.5g

DIRECTIONS:

1. In a saucepan, place the chicken breast, onion, and water to cook over medium heat. Bring the water to a boil. Cook for 10 minutes on low heat with the lid on.
2. Drain the chicken and discard the onion.
3. Cut the chicken and place it in a bowl with carrots, snow peas, peppers, Chinese cabbage, and coriander.
4. In a smaller bowl, combine lime juice, fish sauce, sugar, and chili. Use the mixture to dress the salad. Serve.

40. GREEK SALAD WITH WALNUTS

INGREDIENTS: ✔ VEGETERIAN

- 0.7 oz (20 g) walnut, halves
- 1 ripe tomato, sliced
- ½ red bell pepper, deseeded and chopped
- Pepper to taste
- 1 oz (30 g) low-fat feta, cubed
- ½ tbsp vinegar
- ½ tbsp extra virgin olive oil
- Parsley

- ½ small onion, sliced
- ½ cucumber, halved lengthways, sliced

TIME:
Prep. time: 15 min.
Cooking time: 10 min.
Servings: 2

NUTRITION (PER SERVING):
Calories: 170kcal
Protein: 8g
Cabs: 5g
Fat: 14g

DIRECTIONS:

1. Preheat the oven to 350° F (180° C). Bake the walnuts for 6-7 minutes, until lightly toasted.
2. Set the walnuts aside to cool and chop them.
3. Mix red peppers, tomato, onion, cucumber, oil, parsley, and vinegar in a bowl.
4. Add the walnuts and feta cheese, season with pepper, and serve

41. SPICY SHRIMP LETTUCE WRAPS

INGREDIENTS:

- 1 tbsp lemon juice
- ½ tbsp olive oil
- ¼ tsp honey
- 2 radishes, sliced
- 1 small Persian cucumber, sliced
- ½ head Boston lettuce leaves separated
- 1 tsp grated fresh ginger
- ¼ clove garlic, grated
- Mint and basil for serving
- 1 tbsp Korean hot pepper paste (gochujang)
- ½ lb (230 g) large shrimp, peeled and deveined

TIME:
Prep. time: 15 min.
Cooking time: 13 min.
Servings: 2

NUTRITION (PER SERVING):
Calories: 190kcal
Protein: 36g
Cabs: 13g
Fat: 4.5g

DIRECTIONS:

1. Preheat the oven to 425°F (220°C).
2. Mix gochujang, lemon juice, honey, oil, ginger, garlic, and shrimp in a bowl.
3. Place the contents of the bowl on a baking sheet and cook in the oven for about 13 minutes.
4. Arrange the prawns on top of the lettuce. Garnish with radishes, mint, and basil. Serve.

42. ROASTED VEGGIES AND CHICKPEA SALAD

INGREDIENTS: ✔ VEGETERIAN

- ¼ tsp garam masala
- 8 baby carrots, trimmed and peeled
- ¼ tsp cumin
- ½ red bell pepper, sliced, deseeded
- 0.5lb (200 g) can chickpeas, rinsed and drained
- 0.4 lb (175 g) broccoli, cut into florets
- ¼ cup natural yogurt
- 1.4 oz (40 g) baby spinach leaves
- ½ tbsp lemon juice
- ½ tbsp warm water
- ½ jalapeno, chopped
- Fresh coriander

TIME:
Prep. time: 20 min.
Cooking time: 25 min.
Servings: 2

NUTRITION (PER SERVING):
Calories: 168kcal
Protein: 11g
Cabs: 17g
Fat: 4g

DIRECTIONS:

1. Preheat the oven to a temperature of 400°F (200°C).
2. Mix yogurt, coriander, jalapeno, water, and lemon juice in a bowl. Set aside.
3. Mix cumin, garam masala in a small bowl.
4. Arrange the carrots and the pepper in a baking dish. Next, arrange the broccoli and chickpeas in a second baking dish.
5. Spread the spice mix evenly over all the vegetables and add a drizzle of oil.
6. Roast peppers and carrots for 25 minutes.
7. Roast broccoli and chickpeas for 12 minutes.
8. Place all the roasted vegetables and the baby spinach in a large bowl and gently toss.
9. Drizzle with Jalapeno yogurt and serve.

43. PORK TENDERLOIN, BUTTERNUT SQUASH AND BRUSSEL SPROUTS

INGREDIENTS:

- 1 lb (450 g) pork tenderloin, trimmed
- Salt
- Pepper
- 1 ½ tbsp canola oil
- 1 sprig of fresh thyme
- 1 garlic clove, peeled
- 2 cups brussels sprouts, trimmed and halved
- 2 cups diced butternut squash

TIME:
Prep. time: 15 min.
Cooking time: 30 min.
Servings: 2

NUTRITION (PER SERVING):
Calories: 401kcal
Protein: 44g
Cabs: 25g
Fat: 15g

DIRECTIONS:

1. Preheat the oven to 400°F (200°C). Season the tenderloin with salt and pepper.
2. Heat a pan with a tablespoon of oil over medium heat.
3. When the pan is hot, cook the pork by searing it on all sides. This will take about 8 minutes. Then let the pork rest on a plate.
4. In the same pan, add 2 tablespoons of oil, garlic, and thyme. Finally, add the Brussels sprouts, butternut squash, and a pinch of salt and pepper when the oil is hot.
5. Cook for about 5 minutes, constantly stirring.
6. Put the vegetables in a bounty and arrange the pork on top—roast in the oven for about 15 minutes. Depending on the thickness of the meat, a few extra minutes may be required. You can help yourself with a meat thermometer; the center of the pig needs to reach 140 °F (60°C) to be ready. Remove from the oven and let the tenderloin rest for 5 minutes. Slice and serve with the vegetables.

44. LENTIL CURRY WITH VEGETABLES

INGREDIENTS:

- ½ tbsp madras curry powder
- ¼ cup coriander leaves, chopped
- 130 ml light coconut milk
- 300 g frozen mixed vegetables, partially thawed
- 1 Roma tomato, diced
- 130 g brown lentils, drained, rinsed
- ¼ red onion chopped

TIME:
Prep. time: 15 min.
Cooking time: 30 min.
Servings: 2

NUTRITION (PER SERVING):
Calories: 185kcal
Protein: 11.2g
Cabs: 6.5g
Fat: 26g

DIRECTIONS:

1. To prepare the sauce, mix curry and coconut milk in a deep pan. Cook over medium heat, occasionally stirring until boiling. Add the vegetables that will lower the liquid temperature—Cook with the lid on until boiling. Remove the lid and cook for another 4 minutes or until the vegetables have the consistency that you like.
2. Mix the tomatoes, half of the coriander, salt, and pepper in a bowl to prepare the salad.
3. Add the remaining coriander to the curry. Serve in small bowls with the salad as a side dish.

45. CHICKEN AND ASPARAGUS STIR-FRY

INGREDIENTS:

- ½ tbsp lime juice
- 2 garlic cloves
- ½ tbsp fish sauce
- 1 tbsp low sodium soy sauce
- ⅛ cup low-sodium chicken broth
- ½ lb (225 g) diced chicken breast, 1-inch pieces
- ½ lb (225g) asparagus spears, trimmed and cut into 2-inch pieces
- 1 tsp cornstarch
- 1 tbsp chopped fresh ginger

TIME:
Prep. time: 10 min.
Cooking time: 10 min.
Servings: 2

NUTRITION (PER SERVING):
Calories: 165kcal
Protein: 29.6g
Cabs: 5.5g
Fat: 2.8g

DIRECTIONS:

1. In a bowl, mix lime juice, fish sauce, broth, soy sauce, and cornstarch.
2. With the help of a food processor, blend ginger and garlic until you get a paste.
3. Heat a large skillet over medium heat. When it is hot, you can add the chicken and cook for a few seconds, searing all sides of the meat.
4. Remove the chicken from the pan and let it rest on a plate. Add the ginger and garlic paste to the pan and cook for 2 minutes.
5. Add the asparagus and continue cooking, frequently stirring for another 5 minutes.
6. Add the chicken and pour the lime juice mixture into the pan. Continue cooking for five minutes or more. The chicken must be cooked, and the asparagus should still be slightly crunchy. Serve hot.

46. PB&J OVERNIGHT OATS

INGREDIENTS:

✔ VEGETERIAN ✔ VEGAN

- ¼ cup rolled oats
- ½ cup almond milk
- 3 tbsp peanut butter
- ¼ cup mashed raspberries or raspberry jam
- 1 tbsp toasted almonds
- 3 tbsp whole raspberries

TIME:
Prep. time: 8 min.
(+ 6 hours or more for refrigeration)
Cooking time: 0 min.
Servings: 1

NUTRITION (PER SERVING):
Calories: 460kcal
Protein: 22g
Cabs: 40g
Fat: 32g

DIRECTIONS:

NB. The Peanut Butter & Jelly (PB&J) Overnight Oats is a breakfast that needs to stay refrigerated for at least 6 hours, so it should be prepared the previous day.

1. Combine oats, almond milk, peanut butter, and the mashed raspberries or the raspberry jam in a bowl. Cover and refrigerate overnight for at least 6 hours.
2. In the morning, uncover and top with the fresh raspberries and the almonds.

47. GREEK CHICKPEA WAFFLES

INGREDIENTS:

✔ VEGETERIAN

TIME:
Prep. time: 30 min.
Cooking time: 0 min.
Servings: 2

- ¾ cup chickpea flour
- ½ tsp baking soda
- ¾ cup plain 2% Greek yogurt
- 6 eggs
- ½ tsp salt
- Butter mister

NUTRITION (PER SERVING):
Calories: 414kcal
Protein: 37g
Cabs: 25g
Fat: 20g

DIRECTIONS:

1. Heat waffle iron. In the meanwhile, mix flour, soda, and salt in a bowl.
2. In another bowl, whisk together Greek yogurt and eggs.
3. Pour the whisked eggs with yogurt into the first bowl and stir the ingredients together.
4. Spray butter on the waffle iron. Drop ¼ to ½ cup batter into each section of the waffle iron and cook for up to 5 minutes until golden brown. Repeat with the remaining batter.
5. You can serve the waffles with yogurt, fresh fruits, and your favorite jam, or, if you prefer a savory meal, you can combine them with a light salad. I suggest cherry tomatoes, cucumber, fresh parsley, feta, olive oil, and fresh lemon juice for the salad.

48. EGG WHITE OMELETTE

INGREDIENTS:

✔ VEGETERIAN

TIME:
Prep. time: 10 min.
Cooking time: 10 min.
Servings: 1

- 4 large egg whites
- ¼ tsp of salt
- ⅛ tsp of garlic powder
- ¼ cup chopped scallions - green parts
- Olive oil spray

NUTRITION (PER SERVING):
Calories: 76kcal
Protein: 1g
Cabs: 21g
Fat: 0g

DIRECTIONS:

1. Heat a non-stick pan over medium heat for 2 to 3 minutes.
2. In a bowl, mix the eggs with salt, pepper, and garlic powder until frothy.
3. Add the green onions in the egg whites and make sure they are well mixed.
4. Grease the hot pan with oil and pour the mixture. Tilt the pan if necessary making sure it is evenly distributed during cooking
5. When the egg begins to change consistency, put on low heat and gently and repeatedly lift the corners of the omelet and tilt the pan to allow the still liquid egg to reach the bottom of the pan.
6. When the egg is no longer liquid, gently turn the omelet with two spatulas.
7. After a few seconds of cooking, fold the omelet and serve hot.

49. SCRAMBLED EGG BREAKFAST

INGREDIENTS: ✔ VEGETERIAN

- 1 medium egg
- ⅔ cup egg white
- ½ cup cheddar cheese, shredded
- ½ cup mushrooms, cleaned and sliced
- ¼ of avocado, sliced
- ½ tsp fresh lemon juice

- 1 tsp extra-virgin olive oil
- 1 tbsp fresh parsley, chopped
- Salt and black pepper to taste
- Butter mister

TIME:
Prep. time: 2 min.
Cooking time: 0 min.
Servings: 1

NUTRITION (PER SERVING):
Calories: 203kcal
Protein: 15g
Cabs: 36g
Fat: 5g

DIRECTIONS:

1. First, whisk the egg with the egg whites and season with salt and pepper.
2. Spray some butter on two small-medium size pans and heat it over medium heat.
3. Saute the mushrooms in one pan, cook for 4-5 minutes, then add the parsley and stir. Sprinkle half of the cheese on top of the mushrooms and cover the pan with the lid until melted.
4. Saute the egg in the second pan and let it cook for up to 4 minutes until it's not liquid anymore, then sprinkle the cheese on top of the egg and cover with a lid. Let it cook until the cheese is melted.
5. Plate the egg, the mushrooms, and the avocado in a dish. Season the avocado with salt and drizzle with oil and lemon juice.

50. TURKISH EGG BREAKFAST

INGREDIENTS: ✔ VEGETERIAN

- 2 eggs
- 2 tbsp plain or Greek yogurt
- ⅓ cup red bell pepper, diced
- ⅓ cup eggplant, diced
- ⅓ cup finely chopped yellow onion

- ½ tbsp fresh cilantro leaves, chopped
- 1 whole-wheat pita
- 1 tbsp olive oil
- Pinch each of salt and pepper

TIME:
Prep. time: 10 min.
Cooking time: 10 min.
Servings: 1

NUTRITION (PER SERVING):
Calories: 470kcal
Protein: 23g
Cabs: 28g
Fat: 30g

DIRECTIONS:

1. Heat the olive oil in a large non-stick pan over medium heat. When the oil shimmers, add the chopped onion and cook for 30 seconds until it's translucent. Then, add bell pepper, eggplant and cook for about 7 minutes, stirring occasionally.
2. While the vegetables are cooking, whisk the eggs in a small bowl and season with salt and pepper. When the vegetables are tender, add in the skillet the whisked eggs. Stir and cook until the eggs are softly scrambled and combined with the vegetables.
3. Place the scrambled eggs with the vegetables on a plate, add a dollop of plain or Greek yogurt, sprinkle the cilantro leaves on top, and serve with warmed pita bread.

51. APPLE-CUCUMBER SMOOTHIE

INGREDIENTS: ✔ VEGETERIAN   ✔ VEGAN

- 1 cup apple juice
- ¼ cup unsweetened applesauce
- 1 cucumber peeled and chopped
- ½ lemon juice
- 2 basil leaves - torn
- Ice cubes

TIME:
Prep. time: 30 min.
Cooking time: 0 min.
Servings: 2

NUTRITION (PER SERVING):
Calories: 414kcal
Protein: 37g
Cabs: 25g
Fat: 20g

DIRECTIONS:

1. Blend all ingredients

52. AVOCADO RICOTTA TOAST

INGREDIENTS: ✔ VEGETERIAN

- 1 slice whole-grain bread
- ¼ ripe avocado smashed
- 2 tbsp ricotta
- ½ tbsp extra-virgin olive oil
- ½ tsp fresh lemon juice
- Pinch sea salt
- Pinch black salt

TIME:
Prep. time: 8 min.
Cooking time: 0 min.
Servings: 1

NUTRITION (PER SERVING):
Calories: 290kcal
Protein: 10g
Cabs: 30g
Fat: 17g

DIRECTIONS:

1. Smash the avocado and combine with oil, lemon—season with a pinch of salt and pepper.
2. Toast the bread.
3. Top the toasted bread with ricotta first and then avocado.
4. Serve this toast with scrambled eggs or hard-boiled eggs for a perfect breakfast.

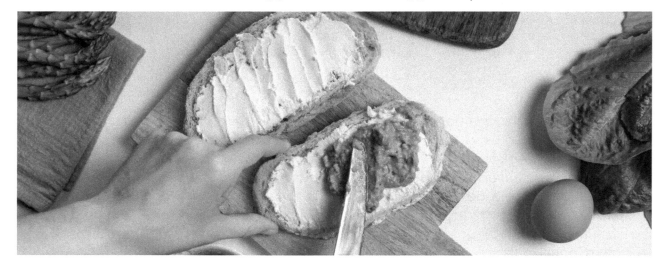

53. GREEN SMOOTHIE

INGREDIENTS:

✔ VEGETERIAN ✔ VEGAN

- 1½ cup unsweetened almond milk
- 2 cups frozen spinach
- 1 cup frozen mango
- 1 medium banana

TIME:
Prep. time: 2 min.
Cooking time: 0 min.
Servings: 2

NUTRITION (PER SERVING):
Calories: 120kcal
Protein: 3g
Cabs: 30g
Fat: 0g

DIRECTIONS:

1. Put all the ingredients in the container of the blender.
2. Start blending on low speed and slowly increase to high.
3. Blend on high speed for 50-70 seconds until the mixture has reached the desired smoothness.
4. Pour the smoothie into glasses and enjoy!

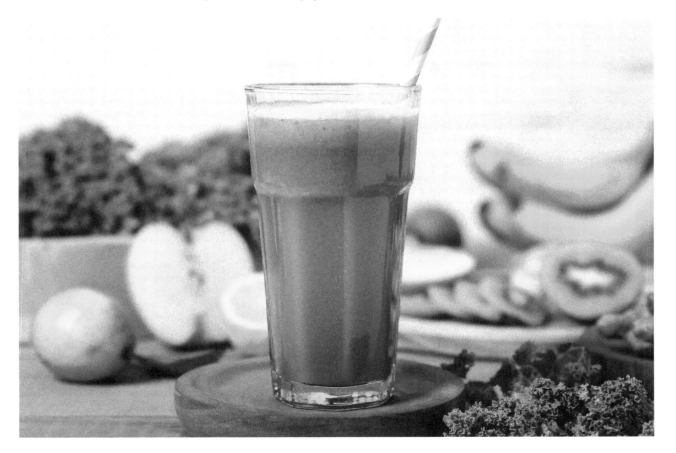

54. APPLE-CUCUMBER SMOOTHIE

INGREDIENTS: ✔ VEGETERIAN   ✔ VEGAN

- 1 cup apple juice
- ¼ cup unsweetened applesauce
- 1 cucumber peeled and chopped
- ½ lemon juice
- 2 basil leaves - torn
- Ice cubes

DIRECTIONS:

1. Blend all ingredients. Serve.

TIME:
Prep. time: 5 min.
Cooking time: 0 min.
Servings: 2

NUTRITION (PER SERVING):
Calories: 76kcal
Protein: 1g
Cabs: 21g
Fat: 0g

55. STRAWBERRIES & WATERMELON SMOOTHIE

INGREDIENTS: ✔ VEGETERIAN

- 2 cups of chopped watermelon
- 1 cup of strawberries
- 1 cup plain low-fat yogurt
- Handful of ice

DIRECTIONS:

1. Blend all ingredients. Serve.

TIME:
Prep. time: 10 min.
Cooking time: 0 min.
Servings: 2

NUTRITION (PER SERVING):
Calories: 149kcal
Protein: 8g
Cabs: 27g
Fat: 2g

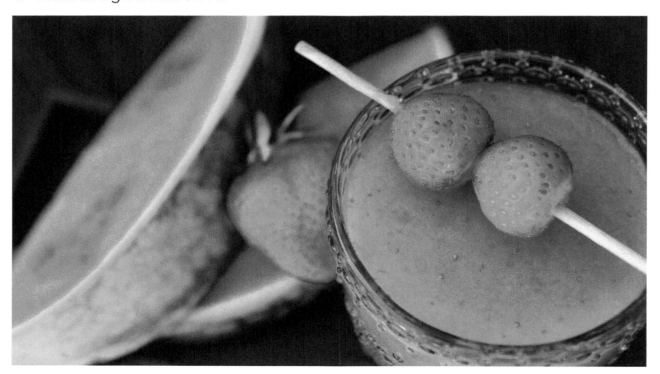

56. SPINACH & STRAWBERRY SMOOTHIE

INGREDIENTS:

✔ VEGETERIAN

- 2 cups of water
- 1 medium banana
- ½ cup low-fat plain yogurt
- 1 cup strawberries, chopped
- 2 cups fresh spinach, chopped

DIRECTIONS:

1. Blend all ingredients. Serve.

TIME:
Prep. time: 10 min.
Cooking time: 0 min.
Servings: 2

NUTRITION (PER SERVING):
Calories: 120kcal
Protein: 4.5g
Cabs: 24g
Fat: 2g

57. MELON SMOOTHIE

INGREDIENTS:

✔ VEGETERIAN ✔ VEGAN

- ½ cup of cantaloupe melon
- ½ cup honeydew melon
- 1 ½ cups of watermelon
- 1 tsp of agave nectar
- Handful of ice

DIRECTIONS:

1. Blend all ingredients. Serve.

TIME:
Prep. time: 10 min.
Cooking time: 0 min.
Servings: 2

NUTRITION (PER SERVING):
Calories: 69kcal
Protein: 1g
Cabs: 18g
Fat: 0g

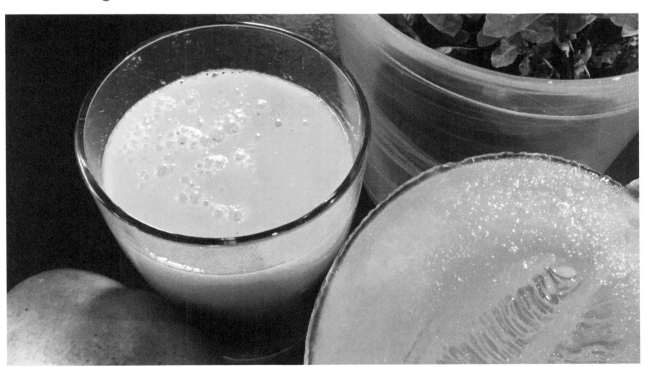

58. CITRUS SMOOTHIE

INGREDIENTS: ✔ VEGETERIAN ✔ VEGAN

- 1 peach peeled and chopped
- 1 orange peeled and chopped
- 1 lemon peeled and chopped
- 2 medium carrots, peeled and chopped

- 1 ½ cup of almond milk
- 5 spinach leaves

TIME:
Prep. time: 10 min.
Cooking time: 0 min.
Servings: 2

NUTRITION (PER SERVING):
Calories: 142kcal
Protein: 4g
Cabs: 29g
Fat: 2g

DIRECTIONS:

1. Blend all ingredients together. Serve.

59. BEET & STRAWBERRY SMOOTHIE

INGREDIENTS: ✔ VEGETERIAN ✔ VEGAN

- 2 cups of unsweetened coconut water
- 2 cups of strawberries
- 1 lime, juiced
- 4 beets pre-cooked and peeled

TIME:
Prep. time: 10 min.
Cooking time: 0 min.
Servings: 2

NUTRITION (PER SERVING):
Calories: 117kcal
Protein: 5g
Cabs: 19g
Fat: 3g

DIRECTIONS:

1. Blend all ingredients. Serve.

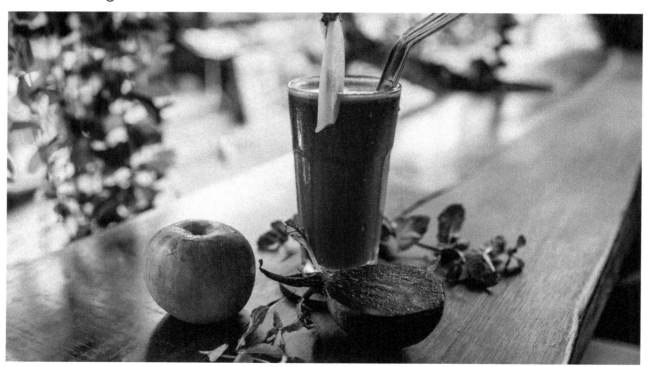

60. FINAL BERRY DETOX SMOOTHIE

INGREDIENTS: ✔ VEGETERIAN

- ½ cup blueberries
- ½ cup seedless red grapes
- ¼ cup ice cubes
- ¼ cup plain low-calorie yogurt

- ¼ cup beet juice
- ½ cup pure tart cherry juice

DIRECTIONS:

1. Blend all ingredients. Serve.

TIME:
Prep. time: 10 min.
Cooking time: 0 min.
Servings: 2

NUTRITION (PER SERVING):
Calories: 140kcal
Protein: 4g
Cabs: 31g
Fat: 1g

61. BLUEBERRY & CELERY SMOOTHIE

INGREDIENTS: ✔ VEGETERIAN   ✔ VEGAN

- 1 cup of blueberries
- 2 celery stalks
- 1 ½ cups of vegan vanilla soy beverage
- Handful of ice

DIRECTIONS:

1. Blend all ingredients. Serve.

TIME:
Prep. time: 10 min.
Cooking time: 0 min.
Servings: 2

NUTRITION (PER SERVING):
Calories: 145kcal
Protein: 4g
Cabs: 33g
Fat: 1g

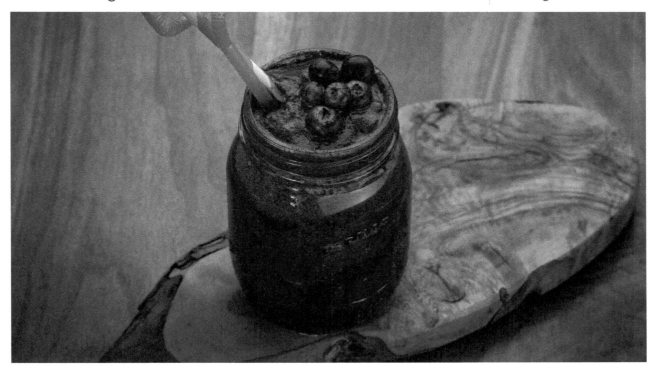

~ CHAPTER 6 ~
# MEAL PLAN

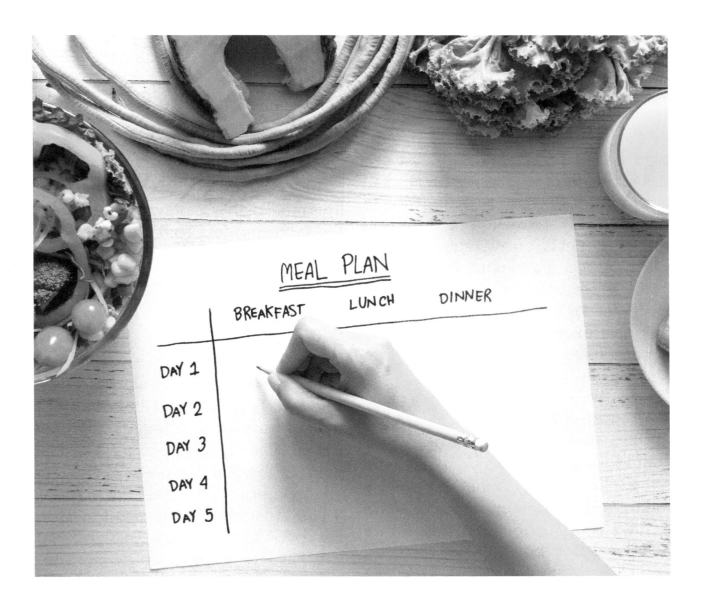

When I said intermittent fasting is a flexible diet and allows you to eat almost anything you want, I wasn't lying. You can consider this chapter as an extra and an accelerator of results. Maintaining a balanced diet will allow you to reach your goals more quickly, but at the same time, not following a meal plan will not prevent you from achieving the results you want, but it will probably take longer.

In this chapter, you will find a meal plan based on a 16:8 diet that can easily be adapted to other variants of Intermittent Fasting. I chose to build this meal plan around the 16:8 method since this diet is, on average, the most used among my clients. In addition, 16:8 represents a good starting point for beginners and a diet that can give excellent results for people already used to Intermittent Fasting.

If you have decided to adopt a rigid portion control and count your macros, the program presented here should be adapted to your personal needs. Indicatively, I tried to build a meal plan that guarantees to consume around 2000 calories per day with a good balance between fat, protein, and carbohydrates.

Unfortunately, due to the limited space available in this book, I have not inserted a meal plan dedicated to vegans and vegetarians. However, I plan to release an add-on for this book with recipes and meal plans dedicated to their dietary needs. In the meantime, in each recipe, I have noted if it is suitable for vegans or vegetarians. I hope this can help you avoid dishes that don't meet your dietary needs and structure your meal plan.

BASIC MEAL PLAN

This meal plan was drawn up assuming the following this 16:8 schedule:

Breakfast - 8 AM
Lunch - 12 PM
Snack - 2:30 PM
Dinner 5:30 PM

These times can be easily altered to suit a 16:8, 14:10, or 12:12 diet. For those who have decided to adopt a 5:2 diet, I will separately include a meal plan for the 500 calorie days you can use to integrate the basic meal plan. If you have decided to use Eat Stop Eat or Alternate Day Fasting, you just have to choose which are your fasting days, and depending on whether you are using a clean or dirty approach, choose whether to do a complete fast or not. As you may have noticed, I specifically left for last one of the most effective and intense intermittent fasting methods. 20:4.

As you have read in previous chapters, this diet carries risks, and I would not feel comfortable building a meal plan for you without meeting you in person. The other diets described in this book allow for some flexibility and margin for error but the 20: 4 diet being extreme requires a precise and meticulous meal plan. For this reason, I have decided to don't provide a meal plan for the 20:4 diet. But, if you want to try it, I invite you to contact a dietician who will create a personalized meal plan for your needs and guarantee your physical and psychological well-being.

In the following meal plan, I have not defined which specific snack to eat each day. Instead, I prefer to provide you with a series of options and let you freely choose the one you like. The main reason is that most variants of Intermittent Fasting are not as strict

as other diets on what to eat even if a well-structured meal plan can act as an accelerator of results.

(*)*Here are some snack ideas:*
- *Fresh fruit*
- *Chocolate protein bar*
- *Fresh veggies mix*
- *Mixed nuts*
- *Greek yogurt and mixed berries*
- *Apple slices with peanut butter*
- *Cottage cheese with flax seeds and cinnamon*
- *Celery sticks with cream cheese*
- *Kale chips*
- *Dark chocolate and almonds*
- *Cucumber slices with hummus*
- *Cherry tomatoes with mozzarella*
- *Chia pudding*
- *Hard-boiled egg*
- *Edamame*
- *Pear slices with ricotta cheese*

	BREAKFAST	LUNCH	SNACK(*)	DINNER
DAY 1	1. Green Smoothie (Recipe 53) 2. Scrambled egg breakfast (Recipe 49) 3. Coffee or Tea	1. Turkey-Walnut Salad (Recipe 12) 2. Two slices of bread 3. Fresh fruit	*Choose one from the list*	1. Sesame-seared Salmon (Recipe 8) 2. Lemony Green Beans (Recipe 14) 3. Fresh fruit
Day 2	1. Green Smoothie (Recipe 53) 2. Scrambled egg breakfast (Recipe 49) 3. Coffee or Tea	1. Mahi-mahi Coconut Curry Stew (Recipe 34) 2. Two slices of bread 3. Fresh fruit	*Choose one from the list*	1. Lemony Green Beans (Recipe 14) 2. Tasty Marinated Tofu (Recipe 22) 3. Fresh fruit
Day 3	1. PB&J Overnight Oats (Recipe 46) 2. Coffee or Tea	1. Stuffed Portobello Mushrooms (Recipe 10) 2. Two slices of bread 3. Fresh fruit	*Choose one from the list*	1. Grilled Prosciutto Wrapped Asparagus (Recipe 1) 2. Mediterranean Roasted (Recipe 17) 3. Fresh fruit
Day 4	1. PB&J Overnight Oats (Recipe 46) 2. Coffee or Tea	1. Cheesy Taco Skillet (Recipe 4) 2. Fresh fruit	*Choose one from the list*	1. Coconut Curried Cod (Recipe 27) 2. Lettuce salad 3. Fresh fruit
Day 5	1. Green Smoothie (Recipe 53) 2. Avocado Ricotta Power Toast (Recipe 52) 3. Coffee or Tea	1. Cauliflower and Ground Beef Hash (Recipe 3) 2. Fresh fruit	*Choose one from the list*	3. Turmeric Sour Cream Tilapia with Parmesan Crust (Recipe 24) 4. Fresh fruit
Day 6	1. Blueberry and Celery Smoothie (Recipe 61) 2. Scrambled egg breakfast (Recipe 49) 3. Coffee or Tea	1. Bolognese Soup (Recipe 11) 2. Fresh fruit	*Choose one from the list*	1. Spinach and Cheese Samosas (Recipe 20) 2. Honey Roasted Baby Carrots (Recipe 16) 3. Fresh fruit
Day 7	1. Blueberry and Celery Smoothie (Recipe 61) 2. Greek Chickpea Waffles (Recipe 47) 3. Coffee or Tea	1. Eggplant Parmesan Panini (Recipe 84) 2. Fresh fruit	*Choose one from the list*	1. Honey Sesame Salmon in Foil (Recipe 32) 2. Lettuce salad 3. Fresh fruit

	BREAKFAST	LUNCH	SNACK(*)	DINNER
Day 8	1. Blueberry and Celery Smoothie (Recipe 61) 2. Greek Chickpea Waffles (Recipe 47) 3. Coffee or Tea	1. Coconut Curried Cod (Recipe 27) 2. Lettuce Salad 3. Fresh fruit	*Choose one from the list*	1. Pork Tenderloin with Butternut Squash and Brussels Sprouts (Recipe 43) 2. Fresh fruit
Day 9	1. PB&J Overnight Oats (Recipe 46) 2. Coffee or Tea	1. Cajun Seasoned Salmon (Recipe 28) 2. Lettuce Salad 3. Fresh fruit	*Choose one from the list*	1. Creamy Garlic King Prawns with Goat Cheese (Recipe 30) 2. Lemony Green Beans (Recipe 14) 3. Fresh fruit
DAY 10	1. PB&J Overnight Oats (Recipe 46) 2. Coffee or Tea	1. Lamb Salad with a Thai style dressing (Recipe 5) 2. Two slices of bread 3. Fresh fruit	*Choose one from the list*	1. Tilapia with Savory Herb Butter (Recipe 25) 2. Lettuce salad 3. Fresh fruit
DAY 11	1. Apple-Cucumber Smoothie (Recipe 51) 2. Avocado Ricotta Power Toast (Recipe 52) 3. Coffee or Tea	1. Turkey Tacos (Recipe 38) 2. Fresh fruit	*Choose one from the list*	1. Zucchini Fritters (Recipe 2) 2. Roasted Orange Cauliflower (Recipe 15) 3. Fresh fruit
DAY 12	1. Beet and Strawberry Smoothie (Recipe 59) 2. Avocado Ricotta Power Toast (Recipe 52) 3. Coffee or Tea	1. Pork Chops with Bloody Mary Tomato Salad (Recipe 31) 2. One slice of bread 3. Fresh fruit	*Choose one from the list*	1. Chicken with Fried Cauliflower Rice (Recipe 37) 2. Fresh fruit
DAY 13	1. PB&J Overnight Oats (Recipe 46) 2. Coffee or Tea	1. Coconut Curried Cod (Recipe 27) 2. Green salad 3. Fresh fruit	*Choose one from the list*	1. Lemon Shrimp in Parmesan Cream (Recipe 26) 2. Lettuce salad 3. Fresh fruit
DAY 14	1. Apple-Cucumber Smoothie (Recipe 54) 2. Scrambled egg breakfast (Recipe 49) 3. Coffee or Tea	1. Pork Tenderloin with Butternut Squash and Brussels Sprouts (Recipe 43) 2. Fresh fruit	*Choose one from the list*	1. Lentil Spinach and Tomato Salad (Recipe 36) 2. Honey Sesame Salmon in Foil (Recipe 32)

	BREAKFAST	**LUNCH**	**SNACK(*)**	**DINNER**
DAY 15	1. Apple-Cucumber Smoothie (Recipe 51) 2. Greek Chickpea Waffles (Recipe 47) 3. Coffee or Tea	1. Spinach and Cheese Samosas (Recipe 20) 2. Honey Roasted Baby Carrots (Recipe 16) 3. Fresh fruit	*Choose one from the list*	1. Chicken and Asparagus Stir-Fry (Recipe 45) 2. Lettuce salad 3. Fresh fruit
DAY 16	1. Beet and Strawberry Smoothie (Recipe 59) 2. Avocado Ricotta Power Toast (Recipe 52) 3. Coffee or Tea	1. Lamb Salad with a Thai style dressing (Recipe 5) 2. Two slices of bread 3. Fresh fruit	*Choose one from the list*	1. Chicken with Fried Cauliflower Rice (Recipe 37) 2. Fresh fruit
DAY 17	1. Apple-Cucumber Smoothie (Recipe 54) 2. Turkish Egg Breakfast (Recipe 50) 3. Coffee or Tea	1. Eggplant Parmesan Panini (Recipe 19) 2. Lettuce salad 3. Fresh fruit	*Choose one from the list*	1. Creamy Garlic King Prawns with Goat Cheese (Recipe 30) 2. One slice of bread 3. Fresh fruit
DAY 18	1. Apple-Cucumber Smoothie (Recipe 54) 2. Scrambled Egg Breakfast (Recipe 49) 3. Coffee or Tea	1. Bolognese Soup (Recipe 11) 2. Two slices of bread 3. Fresh fruit	*Choose one from the list*	1. Chicken with Fried Cauliflower Rice (Recipe 37) 2. Fresh fruit
DAY 19	1. Green Smoothie (Recipe 53) 2. PB&J Overnight Oats (Recipe 46) 3. Coffee or Tea	1. Lamb Salad with a Thai Style Dressing (Recipe 5) 2. One slice of bread 3. Fresh fruit	*Choose one from the list*	1. Sesame-seared Salmon (Recipe 8) 2. Roasted Orange Cauliflower (Recipe 15) 3. Fresh fruit
DAY 20	1. Green Smoothie (Recipe 53) 2. Avocado Ricotta Toast (Recipe 52) 3. Coffee or Tea	1. Lemon Shrimp in Parmesan Cream (Recipe 26) 2. Buttery baked corn (Recipe 18) 3. Fresh fruit	*Choose one from the list*	1. Mahi-mahi Coconut Curry Stew (Recipe 34) 2. Two slices of bread 3. Fresh fruit
DAY 21	1. Apple-Cucumber Smoothie (Recipe 54) 2. Avocado Ricotta Toast (Recipe 52) 3. Coffee or Tea	1. Stuffed Portobello Mushrooms (Recipe 10) 2. Grilled Prosciutto Wrapped Asparagus (Recipe 1) 3. Fresh fruit	*Choose one from the list*	1. Cheesy Taco Skillet (Recipe 4) 2. Honey Roasted Baby Carrots (Recipe 16) 3. Fresh fruit

HOW TO ADAPT THE MEAL PLAN FOR THE 5:2 DIET

If you decided to follow a 5:2 diet, you could modify the meal plan above, replacing two non-consecutive days per week with two 500-calorie days below.

	BREAKFAST	LUNCH	DINNER
500-CALORIE DAY 1	Apple-Cucumber Smoothie (Recipe 51)	Roasted veggies and chickpea salad (Recipe 42)	Spicy Shrimp Lettuce Wraps (Recipe 41)
500-CALORIE DAY 2	Egg White Omelette (Recipe 48)	Tuna and Bean Salad (Recipe 29)	Lentil Curry with Vegetables (Recipe 44)
500-CALORIE DAY 3	Apple-Cucumber Smoothie (Recipe 51)	Asian-Style Chicken Salad (Recipe 39)	Greek Salad with Walnuts (Recipe 40)
500-CALORIE DAY 4	Egg White Omelette (Recipe 48)	Chicken and Asparagus Stir-Fry (Recipe 45)	Lentil Spinach and Tomato Salad (Recipe 36)
500-CALORIE DAY 5	Egg White Omelette (Recipe 48)	Tuna and Bean Salad (Recipe 29)	Lentil Curry with Vegetables (Recipe 44)
500-CALORIE DAY 6	Apple-Cucumber Smoothie (Recipe 51)	Chicken and Asparagus Stir-Fry (Recipe 45)	Lentil Spinach and Tomato Salad (Recipe 36)

∽ COOKING CONVERSION ∼

WEIGHT COVERSION	
½ oz.	15g
1 oz.	30g
2 oz.	60g
3 oz.	85g
4 oz.	110g
5 oz.	140g
6 oz.	170g
7 oz.	200g
8 oz.	225g
9 oz.	255g
10 oz.	280g
11 oz.	310g
12 oz.	340g
13 oz.	370g
14 oz.	400g
15 oz.	425g
1 lb.	450g

LIQUID VOLUME MEASUREMENTS

TABLESPOONS	TEASPOONS	FLUID OUNCES	CUPS
16	48	8 fl. Oz.	1
12	36	6 fl. Oz.	¾
8	24	4 fl. Oz.	½
5 ½	16	2 2/3 fl. Oz.	1/3
4	12	2 fl. Oz.	¼
1	3	0.5 fl. Oz.	1/16

LIQUID VOLUME CONVERSION

CUPS / TABLESPOONS	FL. OUNCES	MILLILITERS
1 cup	8 fl. Oz.	240 ml
¾ cup	6 fl. Oz.	180 ml
2/3 cup	5 fl. Oz.	150 ml
½ cup	4 fl. Oz.	120 ml
1/3 cup	2 ½ fl. Oz.	75 ml
¼ cup	2 fl. Oz.	60 ml
1/8 cup	1 fl. Oz.	30 ml
1 tablespoon	½ fl. Oz.	15 ml

TEASPOON (tsp.) / TABLESPOON (Tbsp.)	MILLILITERS
1 tsp.	5ml
2 tsp.	10ml
1 Tbsp.	15ml
2 Tbsp.	30ml
3 Tbsp.	45ml
4 Tbsp.	60ml
5 Tbsp.	75ml
6 Tbsp.	90ml
7 Tbsp.	105ml

TEMPERATURE CONVERSIONS

CELSIUS	FAHRENHEIT
54.5°C	130°F
60.0°C	140°F
65.5°C	150°F
71.1°C	160°F
76.6°C	170°F
82.2°C	180°F
87.8°C	190°F
93.3°C	200°F
100°C	212°F
110°C	220°F
120°C	248°F
130°C	266°F
140°C	284°F
150°C	302°F
160°C	320°F
170°C	338°F
180°C	356°F
190°C	374°F
200°C	392°F
210°C	410°F
220°C	428°F
230°C	446°F
240°C	464°F
250°C	482°F

∽ CONCLUSION ∽

As you might have discovered from the length of this book, I am a person who prefers to get quickly to the point. Therefore, in these few pages, I have tried to concentrate all the experience I have acquired in my long career to give you a tool that can propel you towards your goals.
After reading this book, you should have understood how intermittent fasting works and the basics of its most famous variants. In addition, you should now have a clearer idea of how to start your diet, some things you will learn along the way, others you will realize their importance later in your journey.

My suggestion is not to try to assimilate all the content of this book in one go; try to start on the right foot and go back to reading the specific sections when you really need them. The path that awaits you is not easy, and a simple book does not have the power to change anyone's life. However, if there is one thing I would like you to make yours after reading this book, it is the idea that "failure is okay!".

There are many super detailed books on incredibly effective diets that could solve all your problems, but only a few of them focus on what I think is essential: "Failure is okay!".
On TV and in the newspapers, we see countless celebrities who have incredible body transformations. But, for them, it is easier! It is very difficult to miss the final goal when you are followed step by step by coaches, motivators, and nutritionists. Well, I can assure you that even celebrities fail or go through difficult times. The thing is, no super-paid coach in the world can put a person back on track when this person thinks they have failed and want to give up.

World-famous dieticians and coaches can not ensure your success. Only one thing that will guarantee you success is your determination and ability to face the obstacles you will encounter during your diet. So, if you have to take only one thing from this book, make sure it is this: set aside the negativity, sense of failure, excessive self-criticism, and start to accept the obstacles you will find as an opportunity to build your path towards the ultimate goal.

Exhale the negativity. Inhale the positivity. Turn your dreams into reality. All the best for a bright future!
- Kat

CPSIA information can be obtained
at www.ICGtesting.com
Printed in the USA
BVHW051612010222
627776BV00006B/947